The Non-stop Lover
and Other Stories from My Practice as a Psychiatrist

by

Dr Magnus Sjögren

Copyright © 2014 Magnus Sjögren

All rights reserved.

ISBN-10: 1502849682
ISBN-13: 978-1502849687

DEDICATION

I dedicate this book to my family, who with their love and support made this book possible, and to the patients who are a never-ending source of inspiration.

CONTENTS

	Acknowledgements	i
	Disclaimer	iii
	Foreword	v
	Introduction	vii
1	The Non-Stop Lover	1
2	The Manic Wall Climber	19
3	The Uninhibited Soldier	33
4	Speed to Overcome Movement	51
5	Twenty Years of Silence	63
6	The Robbing Police	75
7	The Reflex Man	91
8	Shadows Followed Her	107
	About the Author	125

ACKNOWLEDGMENTS

I would like to acknowledge the persons that have been helpful in reading and providing comments on the chapters of this book: my wife, my children, my parents, and then also to other close relatives. Many thanks for your kind support and accurate feedback. Then, thanks goes also to Donna, who edited this book and gave me a lot of valuable feedback and good ideas that made this book better.

DISCLAIMER

The following stories are based on real cases from my practice as a psychiatrist working in the field of psychiatry and neuropsychiatry. However, the names, part of the context, and in some instances the background story, have been modified to avoid any resemblance with the original in order to protect the privacy of the individual. Thereby, any resemblance with real cases is merely coincidental.

Dr. Magnus Sjögren

FOREWORD

The brain is a web of interconnected opportunities; a place where biology, physiology and chemistry meet and generate uniquely human matter; such matter that thoughts, dreams, innovation, drive, love, hate and anger are made of. By controlling our thoughts and emotions, we control the brain. And by controlling and managing physiological and neurochemical processes, the brain controls us. For and within the human brain, there is no reference but us, ourselves, and the world around us. We, along with the world, set the limits and prevent our mind, in the normal situation, from going astray. It is a contextual interdependence that enables this balance. And in view of all the millions of chemical and physiological processes and structural components that work in concert to enable us to maintain this balance and function as humans, it is mind-boggling to think that it actually works at all.

As I hope to convey to you through the stories of this book, there is, however, most often a thin line between harmony and chaos, between function and dysfunction, between normal and disease. Most of the time, our brains do the job for us. But sometimes, and the risk is clear and ever-present, we humans get lost at sea. The following stories are about patients that I have met who somehow got lost. It is my sincere hope that you will find these cases both a good read and a collection of fascinating stories about the brain and its functions. I wish you a good read.

Dr. Magnus Sjögren

INTRODUCTION

Part of your job as a physician is to collect information and make records about observations and findings that you have made. The method of collecting and recording this information is structured and rational, and with the use of a universal language it is aiming at creating a log of information for quick access of relevant medical information. You strive for an efficient language, preferably short sentences, objectivity, and crisp clarity. Any subjective descriptions or statements are discouraged and potentially medically misleading. The text is usually in the shape of prose but actually, it would be better thought of as tables of data which happens to be put into sentences. This format, this language, consequently means that you will read these records with a dry and technical mindset, expecting to quickly get the medical picture, and certainly not expecting to find anything that would arouse your poetic interest. This is all adequate, according to the book and anticipated, simply "lege artis". But the human being behind it is not evident from these technical texts, and when you think of all the stories that are told every day, many times over, it somehow is a loss of human experience. This experience is not relevant for setting the diagnosis or deciding on a treatment, but it is what matters to us as humans. This has, since I started my medical studies, always intrigued me and has driven me to write these stories. My ambition has been to tell a different story: that of the patient.

There are some excellent examples of case stories made into a good read often woven into medical, neurological contexts, for example, as told by Antonio Damasio or Oliver Sacks. Some patients have even made history based on these texts of their astonishing sets of symptoms and signs. Such is the case of H.M., who after surgery of the brain due to severe epilepsy, lost his ability to learn and make new conscious memories. He was stuck in the 1953 baseball series and all that happened before that. He could not build new memories for new events and new facts, and thus everyone that he met from that day on were strangers to him in spite of repeated exposures. The surgery of the brain was done to the hippocampal region bilaterally leading to one of the first observations that this region is vital to learning and recalling information. Another famous story is that of Phineas Gage who, in the mid-nineteenth, century worked as a foreman at a railroad company and who suffered a severe brain trauma causing a confined lesion to the frontal part of the brain. Amazingly, he survived both the accident and the surgery, all taking place in the 1850's, but his life and personality would never be the same again. There are, of course, many more cases, but few reach the patient hall of fame.

The following cases are all from my practice as a psychiatrist. Psychiatry is a practice of the individual. This book is about some of them, for all who want to learn more about the fascinating area of Psychiatry.

THE NON-STOP LOVER

Dr. Magnus Sjögren

1 THE NON-STOP LOVER

According to Maslow, we humans have a relationship with our needs that is bound by a law of nature. The most basic of Maslow's needs are intertwined with life as we know it; they are natural biological processes which, if interfered with, will influence and inhibit essential functions of life. These basic needs are the physiological ones such as breathing, drinking, feeding, staying warm, having sex and sleeping – all of which overlap with the others. For example, lack of sleep will influence our biological systems, and lack of water impacts our chance of survival.

Following those basic needs is a second order of needs which relate to safety. They are not immediately necessary for survival but will become more important after a short time should they fail to be satisfied. Examples of these second-order needs are security of body, health, family, and property.

The third level is about love and belonging. The fourth involves esteem, that is, confidence, respect from others and achievement. Finally, the top level is about self-actualization such as creativity and problem-solving.

One of the absolute basic needs is to be loved. Everyone wants to be loved, or as the poet said, "If not loved, at least admired, and if not admired at least feared" (Hjalmar Söderberg).

Among those of us who live in a prosperous and developed society, there are so many things we take for granted. We seldom take a moment to consider the fact that every day we are able to find shelter, to be fed, to stay warm, and to sleep in a bed. Most of us even take for granted that we will feel loved and have sex, will be respected and seen, and will have an advancing career. Any hindrance to satisfying these needs leads to disappointment and, more often than not, secondary effects such as loss of status.

Some people even go as far as developing and nurturing a

theory to defend why we have it all while others don't, and even why everyone can't have it all. Working within psychiatry and probably within health care in general, it is sometimes ever-so-clear that often there is a narrow line between having it all, being satisfied, and having nothing. The story about the Non-Stop Lover revolves around these needs, but it touches upon them in a different sense, namely what could happen with the Maslovian needs when the underlying biological substrate, the brain, changes. The story is about Charles, a postman who still had it all but somehow lost it.

Charles lived in a small town about 40 kilometres from one of the bigger cities on the west coast of Sweden. He had worked as a postman all his life. He was happy with the freedom he felt, his routines, knowing all about the village, the people and the area in which he lived, mastering all kinds of weather and still delivering the post dry, and doing so most of the year by bike. The landscape surrounding his village was beautiful with the sea and beaches close to his house. There was a small archipelago visible from his kitchen window and his garden was large with several big oak trees and birches. People who commuted to the big city nearby were the ones who loved being able to flee to the countryside every day, perhaps do some surfing in the evening or even sailing, fishing, or just hiking or golfing. The area was once a fishing village about a hundred years ago, but with industrialization also affecting the fishing industry, the little village was almost devoid of people due to urbanisation. Remaining was just a handful of country romantics who took care of the holiday campers and served the local farmers with their recurrent need for extra resources.

But the past 50 years had seen an initially slow change that, in time, would escalate: city folks would return to the countryside as a result of having commuter alternatives. The new train route took merely 30 minutes to bring people to the centre of the big city, avoiding traffic jams and the nuisance of having to drive yourself to work. Charles had experienced most of this change, and the character of his job had to flow with the tide.

Charles' job was to deliver the post in a section of the largest postal area which was by now divided into six sections. When he started to work there in the 60's, there were just two postmen, and it was easy to split the village into two main sections. However, the expansion during the 80's and especially the 90's meant there now had to be six postmen to do the work. Charles had changed his route a few times, and since by now he was close to 60 years of age, he said he appreciated the smaller route for his daily deliveries.

One day the boss, who was fairly new in the village post office, decided to change the route for his post delivery. Charles had to switch from a route on which he had worked for the past five years to another that was new, the reason being that his oldest and dearest colleague was to retire, and it was time to make changes. New staff had been employed, the village was larger, and everyone had to accommodate the changes. All things considered, Charles' boss decided that everyone, including Charles, would have new routes. With Charles' experience, everyone, including Charles himself, assumed that this would work out just fine. It was vetted through and agreed upon.

So the day came when Charles was about to start his new route. Being an early riser, he was the first to arrive at work; he collected his postal delivery package and prepared to leave. As usual, he checked his bike before taking off. No one was given an opportunity to react before it was too late. It turned out that he had started out on the old route, and so his delivery package was all wrong. He didn't seem to bother but delivered post as he felt right. Now, this was peculiar, but perhaps he was just tired. After all, he was over 60 and they had just changed his route. It was a one-time event attributable to human error, and it would all be corrected the next day. At least that was what they all expected, and Charles agreed.

However, when Charles started his route the next morning, he once again took the old route and delivered the post as he felt he should. And it happened again the next morning. Now, this was totally unacceptable. There was a great deal of negative feedback from the locals and intense discussions among his colleagues. Finally, Charles' boss simply could not hold back any longer but started yelling at him, not understanding why Charles kept on doing this.

The only one not reacting was Charles. He seemed to be completely fine with the situation. He was calm and eager to go back to work. To his boss, this was a peculiar response. He had expected him to be sorry, but no: he could not see anything remotely close to the type of reaction he had expected in Charles. How could this be? The fact that he had delivered the post erroneously for three days in a row was a big issue in itself, but the fact that he didn't seem to care was an even greater mystery. Perhaps he didn't understand? Or perhaps he was ill? Or perhaps quietly drunk? Charles just kept acting as if he just wanted to continue delivering to the same route that he had worked for the past 5 years. After some discussion, he was sent home to consider his situation and wait for his boss to call him at home.

A few hours passed before his boss called. Charles had gone home to rest and did not mention anything of this stir to his wife. His boss talked to Charles, and they agreed that he would improve and not continue making any of these serious mistakes. No other change was discussed.

And so Charles went back to his work as usual the next day and made the same mistake once more. This time his boss decided to put Charles back on his old route to see if it worked, and lo and behold, Charles delivered as he used to, and all was well.

As time went on, everything seemed to be fine. However, it didn't take more than three months before Charles had created further confusion in the village. It happened during the spring when there were several red days, or holidays, in a row. The village prepared for some restful days, and the few shops present would be closed. The forecast was telling of ideal weather for sailing or just relaxing by the sea, although it was still too early for any swimming.

But Charles had a different agenda. To him, it didn't matter what season or day it was. On the first of these red days, Charles got up early as usual and rode his bike to work. When he got there, he didn't seem to be bothered about the fact that it was all closed with no prepared post bags to deliver. Instead, Charles collected whatever post he found at the office and created his own bag of post to be delivered that day. Then off he went on his bike for the route he knew so well, having done it on a daily basis for the past 5 years.

Since all of the post was wrongly delivered (and in this small village, the networks were strong), some locals notified his boss the same day. One thing led to another, and Charles spent an hour with his boss later that day in a serious discussion. To his boss' astonishment, Charles acted as if nothing had happened. He was calm – almost indifferent – not reacting to his boss' outbursts, and he oddly repeated that he was eager to go back to work the next morning (which was also a red day). What Charles had done was so strange that his boss decided to suspend him until they had found an explanation and a solution to the dilemma. And so Charles lost the key to the office and was "locked-out".

It was during this time that Charles' symptoms became more noticeable. For the many that knew Charles, it all seemed to develop very rapidly. One day he was fine, and a few weeks later it was very clear that he was almost obsessive in his routines, and that he simply could not, or *would* not, change. He stuck to the same pattern of doing things, such as getting up early in the morning at the very same time each day (regardless of whether it was Sunday or Monday), making breakfast in the same way, selecting the same clothes, walking through the house and the garden along the same paths, and also going to his job every day in spite of him being suspended with no key and no tasks to complete. And every day he was sent back home with the same message: "You are on leave Charles. Take your time to relax".

But Charles *was* completely relaxed. In fact, his mind never considered that he needed any time to relax. He was just eager to do what he sensed he was *supposed* to do, that is, to work. But every day he arrived back home earlier than he used to, and when he got home his wife was about to get dressed and start her breakfast. He greeted her and then went to take a rest, as he always did after work.

When I met Charles the first time, his wife introduced us. It was in the summertime, and Charles was dressed in a shirt, a tie and sports clothing as if he were in between a jogging round and office work. When greeting me, he took off his hat which was a baseball cap. He actually didn't say a word when we were introduced to each other but merely nodded towards me and smiled. It was his wife that gave all the background and talked about investigations that had been done by the general practitioner. They both seemed relaxed, and his wife had a calm expression on her face as if she was relieved to finally be here at the specialist unit in the big city. I got the impression that it had been a stressful time for her and that she now expected to be able to put it all behind her.

Her story about Charles was clear and detailed, only leaving out a few details of their private life. She especially described the changes in his character and the accompanying signs of a disease in such a way that I could just sit back and tick of the boxes in the diagnostic checklist. Obviously, she had a gift of selecting the relevant information and leaving out worries and pain, which I knew she had suffered as well, and which was about to be told in a future meeting with her.

About three quarters of an hour into the meeting, I was left alone with Charles to examine him. As I usually do, I had asked his wife to leave the room in order to have a completely unbiased investigational environment, although I was convinced she wouldn't interrupt. I started out by asking Charles to tell his own story about how he felt. Charles began slowly, speaking in very short sentences and with long pauses in between the words. And although he seemed to smile at me and was very polite, his gestures were limited as was his mimicry. I had to ask him –and in a sense pull the information out of him –rather than his expressing how he felt. Here is an example of how he would answer:

I said, "Please, Charles, may I ask you to describe for me how it all really started for you?"

Charles replied, "I feel fine."

"So, you mean to say that you are well?" I continued.

"Yes," he said.

"What do you have to say about the story that your wife has just told about you and the issues that have arisen in your life?"

"I feel fine."

"Please, Charles, tell me about your work."

"I deliver the post."

"So, how do you do it?"

"I deliver the post by bicycle."

"Yes, you are a postman, and you deliver the post, but how do you do it?"

"I collect the mail, and I deliver the post. I put it in the mailbox."

"Okay, so where do you work?"

"I work in the village."

"How long have you worked there?"

"For many years. I am a postman."

"Have you felt ill in any way?"

"No."

"Your wife told me, and she also told you, that you had some troubles at work. Is that correct?"

"No."

"Well, she explained that you had to change the route, but you didn't do that: you continued with your old route."

"I deliver the post. I am a postman."

"But it happened several times, Charles. You delivered the post to the wrong address because there was a change in your route." (No response from Charles.)

"Can you tell me about it Charles?"

"I am a postman."

"Well, you delivered post to the wrong address, correct?" (No response.)

I brought Charles to the examination room, and he followed gladly. I asked him to take off his shirt so that I could listen to his heart and lungs. He did so without hesitation. He also without any instructions lay down on the investigation bed in order to allow me to test his neurological status, listen to his heart and investigate his abdomen. Then something peculiar happened which relates to what he suffered from. As I prepared to check his pulse, he immediately sat up and reached for my hands and started to check my pulse. He was fully occupied with this activity, and it took him about half a minute to complete the task. He did it flawlessly. So I asked him what my pulse was and he said 100. I said "I suppose that is fine?" and he responded "Yes, it is".

This had happened to me once before: a patient mimicked my profession. This is a sign of their interpreting the context in their perceptual self-centric way. Since it is quite an unusual (but still clear) sign of a frontal lobe dysfunction, I agreed to let him do so. Then I took over again and asked him to help me with my investigation of his cranial nerves. He became an assistant physician supporting me in this.

What I noticed while investigating his cranial nerves and testing the so-called primitive reflexes was that several of these were positive, again indicating a frontal lobe brain lesion. But overall, the neurological and physical status was normal – including his own pulse. The mimicking act has been called the "utilization syndrome" (or Lhermitte's syndrome[1]; not to be mistaken with Lhermitte's sign) and can be described as a loss of one's own frame of reference. Thus, in any given situation, we are all guided by our inner reference base (i.e. experiences, learnt behaviours and preferences) which creates a framework that helps us to select an appropriate behaviour out of a number of options. The outer or external context, (that is, the specific situation with all its environmental cues), provides the guidance to enable an accurate selection of a specific behaviour out of a number of behavioural options. If we lose the inner reference base, we are inclined to be guided completely by external cues, allowing for the possibility of an inadequate selection of behaviour. It may be compared with hypnosis where, upon manipulation, we become disconnected from our inner reference base and act upon instructions. However, with hypnosis the reference base is just temporarily forgotten or de-selected, whereas in the case of a frontal lobe lesion it is gone forever.

It was decided to keep Charles at the hospital for a few days for further investigation. Charles did not object at first, and after having a discussion with his wife (which was more like her describing to him what will happen whilst promising to visit him every day), he agreed to stay. He and his wife followed a nurse to the department while I finished making the records and referrals for investigations of his brain, heart and lungs, which would mean drawing blood and making a spinal tap for investigation of bodily fluids for abnormal patterns, a magnetic resonance imaging of his brain, an X-ray of his chest and echocardiography. To his wife's surprise he did not object but settled right into the department.

At first, Charles was somewhat observant, but he was soon trying to help the nurses and other staff with their daily tasks. He

---

[1] Lhermitte, F. (1986) Human autonomy and the frontal lobes. Part II: Patient behavior in complex and social situations: the 'environmental dependency syndrome'. Ann. Neurol. 19, 335–343

was up early in the morning, and whilst at first he searched the door to the department for a lock to try to get out, he soon went back through the corridor to his room. Afterwards he went to the office where the staff was preparing for the morning routines. Without a word, he helped in all tasks that he was allowed to do, whether it be bringing the breakfast to his fellow in-patients, clearing the tables after a meal, making the beds, or bringing other patients into the department for investigation.

He usually got up early, even before the night shift left, and when he didn't get a task to complete, he kept himself occupied with whatever seemed fitting. He could, for example, move chairs within his bedroom and in the living room to arrange it in different ways; he brought papers that he found to the office; He could also sweep the floor if a broom was available. His actions were characterized by repetitive movements, and he continued these same actions and behaviours every day. He was easily recognized. The routines of the department seemed to fit him perfectly, and he never complained apart from when his wife was about to leave to go home. Then he stood by the door and asked her repeatedly to bring him along as well. But he never became physical – just eager and repetitive. After she closed the door, he stood there for perhaps a few minutes and then went back to his room. If something happened in the department on his way back, he would immediately try to help with whatever task he could.

His way of speaking, whenever he actually spoke, was characterized by short sentences and the use of the same words. The words were elementary and the sentences uncomplicated. He never described anything but seemed fine with the use of a few words to express his needs or to respond. He seemed to understand all that was said to him as he followed instructions correctly. Whenever something happened and he was around, he seemed as calm as ever, never reacting to anything. Even bad words or sad events could not change his temper: he remained calm and unemotional. In fact, something that affected everyone else would not move him at all.

A clear example of his unchanging emotions was when the 9/11 occurred. His wife told about it. Everyone around him was horrified, and there was a lot of discussion. Occasionally, the TV was on and he watched it, but he was completely indifferent. He kept an easy smile on his face, just as always, and he remained calm and positively neutral.

At the hospital we did several investigations: routine blood samples with laboratory analyses of blood cells, blood chemistry including hormones, serology, vitamin B12 and foliate. Magnetic resonance imaging revealed a striking degeneration of the fronto-lateral parts of the cortex, especially on the left side, with a slight widening of the frontal parts of the lateral ventricles. Other parts of the brain showed general age-related changes. This focal, almost confined, degeneration of the frontal parts of the brain indicated a degenerative process which could be a so-called frontotemporal (lobe) dementia[2] or another closely-related degenerative disorder, a rare form of bipolar disorder or schizophrenia, or (very rarely) Alzheimer's disease. Further investigations revealed that his blood flow was decreased in the frontal parts of his brain, and again slightly more accentuated in the left frontal part than the right, while other investigations were all more or less normal (for example, an electro-encephalogram and proteins in the cerebrospinal fluid).

When viewed together, the results of these investigations helped to rule out several common causes of the behavioural changes and diminishing language that was so evident in Charles. The first group of disorders to be ruled out was cerebrovascular disorders (such as post-stroke dementia, multi-infarct dementia, Binswanger's disease, or chronic subdural hematoma) that sometimes may produce such symptoms. Patients with a

---

[2] Snowden JS, Neary D, Mann DM (February 2002). "Frontotemporal dementia". Br J Psychiatry 180: 140–3.

cerebrovascular disorder may occasionally, consistently or intermittently show peculiar symptoms, and it could indicate any type of known brain syndrome.

Although a single infarct or stroke in certain parts of the thalamus[3] occasionally may demonstrate symptoms such as those Charles had, he did not have any signs of vascular disorders. Besides that, there were no signs in the imaging of the brain of any concomitant cerebrovascular changes. Thus, this group of disorders could thereby be ruled out.

The other main disorder to rule out is Alzheimer's disease (AD), or actually Alzheimer-type dementia, since the diagnosis of AD can only be done by a post-mortem investigation of the brain (which seldom is done nowadays). Since AD is a diagnosis that is made by way of excluding other disorders as there are to date[4] no approved positive disease markers, it would be impossible to state with the highest degree of medical certainty that Charles did not have AD. However, since he had signs that rather spoke in favour of another diagnosis, and there were no typical signs of AD, it was ruled out.

According to the brain imaging, Charles did not display any signs of tumours or haemorrhages in his brain. Overall, the lack of any signs indicating other disorders and the typical symptomatology and presence of typical signs made us decide that the diagnosis was most probably frontotemporal dementia.

A few days into Charles' stay at the department, I had the opportunity to speak to his wife alone. We sat down in the physician's office in the department. Charles was unaware that she had arrived, so we were sure he did not search for her, and we could speak uninterrupted. She told me she knew even before he

---

[3] A symmetrical structure connecting many nerve cells, located in the central part of the brain

[4] 15th October 2014

began having trouble at work that something was not completely okay. He had always been a routine person, but about five years ago this had worsened, and he had slowly become more and more rigid and stubborn. She also noted that he spoke less and less, and when the issues at work arose (although it took a few days before she knew), she was not surprised. She had seen the signs at home – the changes in his behaviour and language –but she talked herself into believing they would vanish and he would recover. I asked her about any other changes, and she responded without hesitation that he had shown a clear increase in his drive for sex. It had slowly diminished over time from the vigorous teenage years to a low activity for many years when their kids were still at home. But the past few years had seen a change in that, and when he was about 58, his appetite had increased again.

At first, Charles' wife thought it was an age-related crisis: they were both near 60. But with the other changes in his life, she interpreted his behaviours as a sign of something else. She thought that perhaps he was depressed or confused. Perhaps life was challenging to him and perhaps he was in search of something more meaningful. He seemed hungry for love, and so she wanted to comfort him and decided to give it to him. In the beginning he was caring and responsive, and they both seemed to enjoy it. For a while she even thought that they had the best time of their life together. But then eventually, as his need seemed to increase, she felt it was a bit too much for her, and she had to find ways to decline in a respectful way. Charles was rather easily managed, but at times he could insist and become physically dominant – although never abusive. His wife had to give in more and more often, but then he sometimes seemed to accept her refusing him.

Charles seemed to become more and more demanding – or was it that his need was increasing? His wife wasn't sure. She started to develop routines to avoid him such as taking walks outside and visiting friends. She could manage to avoid his appetite (especially during the morning hours) by being active and staying outdoors or away, but at bedtime it was more difficult. At the same time, his diminishing language made what he really meant and wanted confusing to her. They had always talked a lot to each other, at least she to him, but when he suddenly began demonstrating such a growing appetite for her (and for sex in general), she could not use her words to calm him down or keep him away. What had been a pleasure for them both in the beginning turned into a game of hide and seek – not for fun, but to avoid him, and the hunt was becoming a terror.

His wife had to increasingly make use of various tactics and went as far as to hit him where it hurt the most; still, he did not change. He seemed to be programmed for sex, and she was to be the victim since she was his partner for life. The situation finally came to a head when she had to lock herself in whilst he was searching for her in the garden. She had planned it for a while, and she developed a routine of luring him out into the garden before they had sex. Then, when all doors were locked without him knowing it, she returned back to the house and locked the front door. She watched him from another window as he worked at trying to open the door. Somehow, he just continued without letting go and without giving any sign of frustration or emotion. He just continued to try to open the door for perhaps an hour and a half, after which he began walking about outside to search for her again.

Charles' wife felt terrible the whole time for not letting him in – especially since it was somewhat cold outside (being it was in the autumn). She kept Charles locked out for about an hour more until she sensed that his hunger had calmed down. When she opened the door, he just entered without a word or any sign of anger and walked straight to the television and sat down to watch.

This game continued for a few months almost on a daily basis. His routine of walking outside everyday helped, and as the winter approached his drive seemed to be more tolerable due to the influence of a lower temperature, as his drive faded faster. In the coldest months she only had to lock him out for about 15 minutes or so. He never got upset, but he just continued to try to open the door. During the worst period of Charles' obsessive behaviour, his wife had to lock him out twice a day and still be prepared for encounters at bedtime. This behaviour went on for about a year until she developed several ways to avoid his advances. She then managed to keep them at a lowest possible frequency, which meant a few times per week. After a year it also seemed that his sexual behaviour had changed somewhat. Originally, they had good, interactive sex, but with time Charles became more and more ritualistic and behaved like a robot just repeating the same movement over and over until he was done. All the while he did not say a word. Finally, after about one or two years, Charles had other signs of an illness, and his mental inflexibility and lack of creativity took over, making it easier and easier for her to keep the frequency down. By then she had long since understood that something was wrong with his behaviour. Still, his drive for sex never changed.

So what then was really wrong with Charles, and why did he develop this strange behaviour? When viewed together, the signs, the symptoms, his behaviour, the progressive nature of the disease, and the sum of all the investigations clearly revealed that he had a neurodegenerative disorder with a frontal focus, such as in frontotemporal dementia. There were no signs of any other disorder except for a primary degenerative disease. Primary means that it affects the brain cells at first. By impairing the functioning of the brain cells it successively leads to focal cell death, which spreads to affect larger brain networks, leading to detectable symptoms and clinical dysfunction, later to complete loss of function, in that order. Anatomically, as visualized by brain imaging, it step by step breaks down the structures of the brain.

In the beginning, disorders such as frontotemporal dementia may mimic other disorders, and it is common to interpret the symptoms as signs of a crisis, a mood disorder or psychosis. The presence of changes in the brain as detectable by brain imaging supports the diagnosis, but the signs are not specific. The progressive nature of the disorder often makes it easier to diagnose using repeated investigations over time. Charles deteriorated over time and more or less completely lost his ability to speak. Overall his expressive communication also diminished leaving behind a wordless and empty gaze. However, he continued to react adequately to verbal instructions for many years into his disorder. Even when the disorder had broken down his abilities to walk and move about, when he was bedridden and vegetative, he still reacted to spoken language and seemed to try to follow what was said to him. His drive for sex was only directed towards his wife and he never stimulated himself as far as we know. This drive diminished as well, although when his wife turned up, even in the later stages of his disease, he could occasionally still make sexual passes and movements towards her.

How could we explain his behaviour as anything more than that which is typical of a neurodegenerative process in the frontal areas of the brain? And what was behind his increased drive for sex and his language changes? The sexual behaviour has been explained by some scientists as being due to a brain lesion in the central parts of the cerebrum (such as the hippocampus, the temporal lobes, and hypothalamus). It may be seen when one or both of the temporal lobes are affected, such as in the Kluver-Bucy syndrome[5]. It may sometimes be related to a change in the activity of the fronto-subcortical, or meso-limbic pathways, which are mostly innervated by dopaminergic neurons. It has also been

---

[5] Adel K. et al. (1998). Functional Neuroanatomy. McGraw-Hill. "The Kluver-Bucy syndrome is a clinical syndrome observed in humans and other animals after bilateral lesions in the temporal lobe that involve the amygdala, hippocampal formation, and adjacent neural structures.

identified in patients with other dementia disorders, such as bipolar disorders, when there seems to be an over-activity in these brain areas. Broca originally described the overall syndrome with deterioration of spoken language in the 19th century[6]. He ascribed the importance of the left frontal brain to the generation of spoken words. Usually, one speaks about Brodmann Area 44[7] as the centre for the generation of spoken language, and any lesion or change that impacts this brain area will, to some extent, influence our expressed language. It may also go beyond spoken language to other areas where our language is imperative for the internal guidance of our behaviours.

In view of his increased drive for sex and his increasingly stereotyped sexual behaviour and manners overall, we may ask if Charles felt pleasure, and if so, was it felt in the same way as in a non-affected individual? Philosophically speaking, this question probably could not be answered with preserved scientific objectivity: obviously, we did not then and do not now have Charles as a source of this information. What we can say is that he most likely did feel pleasure, since the mechanisms behind pleasure are universal to mammals.

To give some background on this, we have to go back to studies done by Peter Milner who investigated how rats responded to weak electrical stimulation. Milner found that there are some regions in the brain that, when electrically stimulated, give rise to pleasure leading to addiction[8]. Other regions give rise to pain, leading to avoidance. It is known that individuals with this type of disorder also have changes in a neurochemical system called "the

---

[6] Dr. Paul Broca". Science 1 (8): 93. August 21, 1880

[7] http://en.wikipedia.org/wiki/Brodmann_area_44

[8] Liebowitz, Michael, R. (1983). The Chemistry of Love. Boston: Little, Brown, & Co.

dopaminergic": this system is the same as the one that is responsible for pleasure, lust, and drive and is amenable to addiction. Brain structures such as the ventral tegmentum[9] and the nucleus accumbence are core components in this dopaminergic system, and changes in them would most probably be the reason underlying the symptoms and the drive that Charles displayed. The brain imaging done could not tell if these systems were changed since these are both small and located deep down in the centre of the brain: the routine investigations would not reveal these specific changes.

Another typical behaviour that Charles showed was inflexibility, which later evolved into stereotypia, as exemplified by his extreme routine behaviour. This has been linked to degeneration or changes in the anterior cingulate cortex[10] and to changes in the fronto-subcortical pathways (that is, the ones that are innervated by dopaminergic neurons) and to changes in the larger frontal brain network involving both the dorsolateral prefrontal cortex as well as the orbital frontal brain and subcortical structures, including those that are part of the dopaminergic system.

As for Charles, he was blessed with not seeming to care. In spite of all that happened to him, he just kept on, never reacting to anything. And although his wife managed to avoid an overdose of his sexual behaviour, as long as he lived his inner drive for her was non-stop.

---

[9] http://en.wikipedia.org/wiki/Ventral_tegmental_area

[10] http://en.wikipedia.org/wiki/Anterior_cingulate_cortex

2 THE MANIC WALL CLIMBER

Sander was forty-two when I first met him at a psychiatric ward in Sweden. His hair was wild and slightly grey. His gaze was intense, and his movements were fast and ever-changing. He had arrived at the psychiatric emergency unit voluntarily, accepting the proposal of his daughter to go there for a medical examination. For several nights he had been up walking about in the house, talking nonsense, disturbing the sleep of others, especially his daughter, who temporarily lived at home with him. At the unit he caught everyone's attention by screaming and shouting, giving orders to both patients and staff, and switching rapidly from grandiose manners to nervousness and stale laughter. His daughter, who was eighteen years old and studied at the local high school, briefly introduced him. She said that he was a construction engineer and divorced. She was his only daughter.

For about a month Sander had been sleeping poorly. He had been up walking and talking through each night. At first it was only for about one hour, but after a few nights it escalated, and in recent days he was up almost all night, not even sleeping in the daytime. He seemed to grow more and more restless, so at work they had told him to take some time off. His boss made an appointment for him with a physician, but Sander did not turn up. His boss then decided to pay him a visit at home, and it was then that he met the patient's daughter and described to her the situation at work. After this meeting with Sander's boss, she decided to take her father to the hospital. She told me that Sander was much appreciated at work and that he enjoyed his work. She said that there was nothing in his work situation that possibly could explain this change in behaviour. She also cited his boss as giving much support to Sander and wishing him well.

His daughter did not know if he had been ill before, but she remembered that when her parents divorced he was upset and could not work for at least a month. She was seven years old at that time and had vague memories of the event, but clearly recalled him being up at night. Then she recalled another event a few years later when she spent time at her mother's place for longer than usual since it was said he was on a business trip abroad. She recalled that she found this strange due to the fact that he never had done something similar before, and no one ever talked about his trip before or after he went away. Since Sander's parents were both deceased and he had no brothers or sisters, there was little information to be gathered about his childhood except from Sander himself. The daughter recommended we talk to her mother about Sander, although she clearly indicated they had not spoken for several years and that she had been brought up by her father.

Sander's daughter mentioned that during the last few nights she had tried to talk to her father to try to understand what was troubling his mind. It was then she noticed that he seemed to talk mostly to himself about things that happened many years ago and also about new topics that she did not recognize at all. He had talked, for instance, about selling the house and buying an apartment, which upset her a lot. They got into a brief quarrel, and since she did not understand the logic in his reasoning she had asked him if he really was serious about his plans. When she questioned him being serious, he began yelling at her, saying that she cost too much and that he could not afford her. Then he immediately began to cry briefly, and then quickly began talking about bugs eating away at the foundation of the house. He feared that he and his daughter may end up "in the mud" if they did not do something about the situation.

Sander's daughter was so stunned by this sudden change in the discussion that she became completely silent. He continued to quickly move into another topic (which she was too upset to remember), but it had nothing to do with the cost or the state of the house. After her being silent for a while, she slowly came out of her state of astonishment, but she did not respond to his monologue. He began murmuring quietly, almost as if he was no longer talking, but just making noises that sounded like words.

Bit by bit Sander's daughter started realizing that he displayed signs of being mentally ill. The thought of him being out of his mind scared her at first, but with the escalation of the situation and his walking around murmuring to himself, she realised that there was no time to mourn, and she needed to do something. She had already toyed with the idea of taking him to the hospital, but now she moved into action trying to convince him that it was the best thing to do. After several hours, perhaps three, he finally gave in. So she ordered a taxi and prepared him to go. It took her a while to convince him to wear a jacket, even though it was autumn and pretty cold outside. When the taxi arrived, it turned out that the driver had been used to similar situations, so he immediately started to help Sander's daughter bring him to the waiting taxi. The driver didn't need any direction. He said, "I know where we are going," and off they drove into the dark towards the psychiatric emergency unit.

Sander's first examination at the unit was difficult to complete since he was restless and wanted to leave the room. He didn't finish any conversations, and he refused to answer to any questions from the psychiatrist. Before he left the room he stated that he had "agreed to a physical exam, but not this" (not clarifying what "this" referred to). He more or less ran out of the examination room and thereafter stormed about in the corridor trying to find a way out, complaining loudly. Since his daughter had stayed with him in the examination room to try to keep him calm, she carefully kept trying to convince him that this was the best thing for both of them. After at least an hour, her convincing seemed to do the trick. He accepted a brief physical examination of the lungs and heart, and afterwards he also asked for an examination of the abdomen.

Meanwhile, the examining psychiatrist began to ask Sander a few questions:

"Sander, how have you slept for the past few days?"

Sander replied briefly, "Fine."

"Have you had any pain?" the psychiatrist continued.

"No."

"Any nightmares?"

"None."

"How about stress? Are you feeling uneasy about anything?"

"I feel great – perhaps even the best in my life!" Sander assured him. The responses were so short they could have set a record in speed talking.

The psychiatrist thought for a moment and then asked, "Why do you speak with such a rapid and loud voice. Are you angry?"

Sander replied, "NO, I am not angry!" as he gestured with his hand. Then he added, "Can I leave now?"

"I'd like you to stay for additional examinations and to ensure that you get some sleep," the psychiatrist said.

Sander did not refuse, but simply said, "I feel fine."

As the Psychiatrist did not want to violate any laws, he explicitly repeated, "I'd really like for you to stay."

Sander then responded, "My daughter wants me to."

Since such a response cannot be regarded as explicit consent, the physician repeated the question, "But I'd like to know if you yourself will agree to stay and undergo further examinations and possibly treatment?"

Sander practically shouted, "Yes, yes, yes! I will stay!"

Sander followed a nurse and his daughter to a psychiatric ward to get him settled in. It was close to five a.m., and there wasn't much activity going on in the corridors and meeting rooms of the hospital. The only sounds that could be heard were the flushing of water in the tubes, some distant steps from night staff walking from a department to the lab or the radiology unit, and Sander's singing, which really was a mixture of songs, most of which he knew only in part. He never really finished any song but jumped from tune to tune, from key to key, sometimes jumping and skipping in the middle of a refrain. His voice was soft and sometimes quite beautiful, but he interrupted his singing with impulses of high-pitched noises, and bursts of shouts, and even laughter, which all seemed like something taken from a comedic horror movie.

Just before he arrived at the door of the department (while still being in the hallway), he turned around and started running in the opposite direction. But only after a few steps he stopped himself and began walking back in a dramatic manner to his daughter and to the door of the department saying that he "did not feel like running tonight, but it is more fun being with you," not specifying whom he referred to. The attending nurse's pulse had gone from 70 to 150 in a few seconds as she had prepared to call for help and run after him. Slowly, perhaps with a few "skipped" heart beats, her rhythm returned to normal.

Sander's first few days in the department were characterized by his restlessly walking back and forth in the corridor and stopping to have a conversation with other patients, only to end it after a few lines. Some of the other patients complained about his offending them verbally and that he kept them awake at nights. He slept only about one or two hours a night before he agreed to try medicine: an anti-psychotic and a sleeping pill. He talked about different projects that he had in mind, some of which he had already started and others which he was about to initiate. The projects involved areas such as engineering and construction, starting an online casino, getting married again, taking dance lessons for Finnish tango, and rebuilding the houseinto a Medici villa, although he never again mentioned the bugs that were about to tear it down. When asked about them he only said that they were gone.

Sander tried to engage other patients at the ward in his projects, but only a few agreed to join him, and eventually only one partnered up with him and discussed for hours how to execute these various projects. The one idea most vividly and frequently talked about was the construction of a new bridge across the channel in the city. He drew up models, once even on the wall paper, and made calculations over and over again. A close examination of these drawings and calculations showed that they all had an excellent beginning, but they seemed to stop half-way through and were never finished.

During his first few nights in the department, Sander managed to pee in one of the larger plants, start a short track race in the corridor, make exclamations from famous poets, describe how he would rob a bank and start lending for a lower rate than any existing bank today, tell about his love affairs with different women and claimed he was an attractive man to other men, although he stoically had refused any such invitations. He also went into other patients' rooms on two different occasions, suggested that he was a great lover and proposed that they sample his skills. But nothing ever happened: his invitations were all refused. For a few nights, the staff on night shifts saw their working hours fly by ever so fast being busy with following him and keeping an eye on his adventures.

In one of our first meetings, Sander and I started to discuss treatment options. He said he was interested, but he kindly and very "warmly" refused. During our discussion I mentioned lithium, which is an effective treatment for acute manic episodes, as an option. In spite of it being such an effective treatment, lithium is also associated with "madness" in the general population, and when I offered this treatment to him, he not only declined but also stretched his neck and looked at me with strange, staring eyes, as if I were offering a medieval form of torture, and said, "Dear Dr Sjögren, again, I decline." After our meeting he told everyone in his vicinity, "I'm not mad at all, and I don't want to be treated as such". Therefore, the only treatment he had accepted was a daytime sedative, a sleeping pill at night, and after two days, anti-psychotic medication as well.

Thus, after a few "stormy" initial nights, Sander successively became slightly tired and then struggled to continue talking and moving about at the same pace as he had done for the past few weeks. As this is an important phase in the treatment of a psychotic person, we took care to observe his ability to control his movements since he might have lost his balance. Sometimes there is a drop in blood pressure, and if that were the case, he could hurt himself. These "side effects" set-in at the same time as the anti-manic effects occur.

When Sander saw me approaching him in corridor and knew that I wanted to talk with him, he immediately approached me and said, "Finally, some help!" stretching out his arms as if he wanted to hug me. So I accepted the hug and asked him if I could help him in any way. He said, "Yes, of course great Master Doctor," but then he dramatically changed his posture and attitude. He continued with, "But you of all people should know how to help me." So I asked him if it was the treatment that he meant was helping him, and he replied in a rather loud voice, "Yes everyone can see that" and extended his arms from his body taking a pose as if he was a proud Matador. Then he continued to ask, "Now, help me to get in contact with my daughter, because she and I need to talk about my life and all that."

So what continued was a discussion which went back and forth between logic and facts based on his interpretation of the situation, which still was somewhat distorted. He seemed to want to make some decisions about whether to leave the department or not, whether to change the treatment or not, and what else we could do to help him. Before we had finished the discussion, or at least when I came to a point where I had felt that we were approaching some conclusions, he suddenly ran as quickly as he could manage away from me in the corridor.

We did not speak again for the next two days due to my being assigned to other tasks, mainly, the emergency unit. When I came back two days later he again approached me and said, "Thank you sublime existence for coming back." Then he added, "You have already saved me thank you so much," and then he went down the corridor singing a made-up song about "great Master doctors". I noticed that although he used the same words as before, he moved at a slower pace and his face seemed to look somewhat brighter. Furthermore, he did not speak continuously, and he did not engage in everything that happened around him, which were clearly signs of improvement.

After three days Sander was allowed to go out for a walk with a staff companion. When he reached the courtyard, he immediately noticed some trellises for plants that were leaning against the wall. He very quickly began to climb the wall of the building, which was about eight metres high, and he didn't stop until he had reached the top. There, on top of the house, in front of the whole hospital, he started to sing some of his favourite tunes, constantly interrupting himself to change the tune and sometimes to cheer for himself. This caused a lot of stir, and the staff member called upon others to help him with this patient who seemed enthused about all the action happening on the ground. He probably could have stayed there for as long as he liked since it turned out that the fire door to the roof was locked and jammed, and no one could come up to help him get down to the ground. However, instead (and quite characteristic of the state of mind he was in), he started to climb down the trellis to the ground, all the while singing his favourite tunes triumphantly with a loud and clear voice.

It was about a week later before he was let out again. He had spent the whole time inside due to the possibility of recurrence of what was deemed to be high-risk, potentially self-destructive behaviour. There were signs of him getting better, and he apologized for his behaviour several times as he explained that it was due to him being "hypnotized and struck by a magic spell". He had asked almost every day about being allowed to get some fresh air outside, so we decided to try again. Overall, his sleep was improving, he was eating more regularly, and his agitated speech also had reduced substantially. Eye contact and conversation improved, and so we decided that we would try to take him for another walk outside.

The plan in situations like this is always to first reduce the signs and symptoms of the disorder to reduce any risk of harm, and then, when there's a clear clinical picture of an overall improvement, to start introducing exposure to the individual's normal life, his habits, his social network and after a time of recovery, finally his job. At the same time, the aim is to stabilize and then when the patient is back to his habitual status, reduce the dosages of various medications. Therefore, attempting again to expose Sander to a walk in the park outside was a natural part of the plan. This time Sander would have two guardians walking next to him to prevent him from climbing up a tree or a building. We also talked to him about his risky behaviour, and he assured us several times that he would never do this again. So he was let out with the two guardians.

It was a Thursday afternoon from what I recall. The weather was fine with a typical autumn temperature and a few clouds in an otherwise-clear sky. It was an excellent day to be out and stroll in the park. Sander was cheerful that he was going out, but at the same time he also complained a few times before reaching the door that he had been inside for a whole week without being let out. The guardians were well-prepared: both were male, pretty strong, and viewed the task as a positive challenge. They had even bragged about their previous experiences in the morning briefing and claimed nothing would happen with them being around. The guardians themselves talked to Sander giving him instructions about how to behave outside. And so they were let out of the department.

They took a few steps out into the front yard of the psychiatric unit and into the beautiful weather. Sander was delighted and suggested they walk towards a green park and since this already was the plan, so they did. Sander said that he was the happiest man alive. He continued that he appreciated their generosity and companionship. But he didn't stop there: he flattered the guardians, telling them how strong they were and how safe he felt in their company telling them how much everyone respected them. Somehow this positive and perhaps valuable talk (and perhaps also his continuous generation of words, which for once seemed to make sense at least to the guardians) distracted them. According to what they told afterwards, their attention faded only slightly, but it was enough to give Sander an opening.

The guardians claimed that it all happened so quickly. At one moment Sander was praising them and the next he was gone. They claimed it felt inadequate to lock him up into their arms, which would have seemed as though they were restraining him – a sort of repeal which would have been unethical and contra-therapeutic. And so Sander was once again on the loose, and again he faced the very same building that he had climbed just a week before. He started to climb the trellis and was once again on the roof in a matter of less than a minute.

There he stood once again at the top with his arms raised straight up in the air, his eyes facing the sky, singing his favourite tunes –this time Swedish dance songs. Perhaps his singing was better now, his tone more accurate, his rhythm more steady, and perhaps he finished more songs compared to last week. Once again the alarm bell went off, and we ran outside to find the two embarrassed guardians standing there looking at the roof.

The view of him standing on top of the building singing was terrifying, and we all (especially the two guardians) felt embarrassed for this having happened again. This time, however, we were better-prepared, and we knew how to get him down to the ground. The fire staircase had been fixed, and one of the guardians was already heading in that direction and began to run up the stairs. When Sander heard that someone was approaching, he decisively started to climb down the same way he went up. He was real steady and looked like an experienced climber, which wasn't very surprising, and came down in what seemed to be less than a minute. When he reached the ground, we were there waiting for him, and without much talk we walked him back to the department. We felt ashamed, inferior as professionals. Sander was happy as a bird.

At the debrief we felt that we had failed in judging his mental state and decided to be even more attentive than before. We introduced twice-daily assessments of his status and decided to keep the medication at a high enough level to ensure that his manic symptoms would decrease. Although we were set on enabling a swift recovery, it took yet another couple of days before he was let out for a walk again. This time when he was led out, he had two even more-cautious guardians who took him straight from the department by car to an open field where there were no buildings or trees around. There he spent two hours every day for the next two weeks, and it was clear that he enjoyed and benefitted from it. With this strategy he gradually improved, and after about two weeks we were able to reduce his medication and remove the guardians.

Approximately ten days later, Sander gave me permission to speak to his ex-wife. I got her contact information from his daughter and gave her a call one afternoon. Her story gave additional information that confirmed our notion that Sander was suffering from a Bipolar Disorder. When they met, he was very charming and had a lot of energy, and she immediately fell in love. They were quite young, and she was impressed by his physical stamina and his wide interests. These interests, she was to find out after about a month or two, gradually diminished a bit, and Sander became what she described as more normally interested in everyday things which also included their relationship. She never had any thought that it could be a sign of illness, but she saw it more as enthusiasm induced by being in love – a very normal reaction. It didn't take long before their love for each other was established, and they developed a relationship. When they began living together, perhaps after a year, there was a period in their relationship where he seemed to once again escalate and engage in different activities, speak loudly and fast, and sleep just a few hours per night. Since they both were studying at that time, she interpreted it as him being stressed over attempting to do well in his University studies.

It wasn't until about two years later when Sander developed symptoms of a mild but lasting depression that she started to think about his mental state. It began with tiredness and low energy and evolved into self-complaints, low self-esteem, a sullen mood and discussions about death. He also stopped eating for a while and had difficulties concentrating on his work. She then decided to take him to a physician, and Sander was diagnosed as suffering from depression. The doctor initiated anti-depressive treatment, which was the turning point. After about four weeks Sander had improved, and after two months he was back to his habitual self. Their life together returned to normal, and the affection that they felt for each other was even further strengthened after this episode.

But their relationship would be challenged once more: it was only about one year later that Sander developed a manic episode, and things started to get completely out of hand. Within a couple of weeks he escalated his tempo, became hyperactive, spoke non-stop, didn't sleep, and engaged in several of projects that were never finished. He also spent a lot of money and went out partying. Once, his wife even suspected that he initiated new relationships with other women. He may have even tried drugs during that period.

Everything came to a halt when the police brought him back home after a stormy night out. Since he was both wild and angry, they took him to a psychiatric unit, and he was treated. After a few weeks, he recovered. But this would not be the end: he had yet another episode shortly after the birth of their daughter. But the change in their relationship had already started before her arrival (probably with his wild life during the last manic episode), and was it not for all the relational mending and fixing that was going on at the same time it would soon have led to a separation. Sander's ex-wife explicitly stated that she could not endure his mood swings and his behavioural changes: they would inevitably continue. It all was too unpredictable for her to withstand in the long run. And so, after a few years they broke up. Their daughter stayed with her mother for a few years. After that she then split her time between her father and mother. When her mother started to date a new man, she tended to spend more time with her father.

Sander improved and was soon let out of the hospital. He eventually returned to his job and regained his former stability, this time supported with lithium treatment. He remained stable for several years, and his network, including everyone from his daughter and boss to his friends, set up a support system that made it easier to identify early signs of illness. Sander had come to terms with this, and for as long as I followed him, he remained healthy.

Bipolar disorder, or commonly also called manic-depressive disorder, is a mental illness classified as an affective or mood disorder. It affects about four per cent of the population and is (as was the case of Sander) characterized by episodes of a hyperactive mood known as mania alternating with episodes of depression. The gender distribution is equal, and genetic factors have been found to contribute to the development of the disorder. The severity of symptoms may vary within an individual, such as between episodes, and the symptoms are also differentially expressed between individuals. In the worst cases, psychosis may prevail.

It is important to be aware that bipolar disorder may involve severe manic episodes with challenging and stressful behaviour replaced by depressive episodes with suicidal ideation. The consequences of bipolar disorder are also extensive with social stigma and prejudice against the affected and suffering individuals. Sander had most of these symptoms and suffered a lot of the consequences in-between his episodes. He was fortunately respected at work and managed to have an effective social network, especially a strong relationship with his daughter. One thing brings this story to a full circle: Sander's behaviour during his manic episode involved him starting a lot of projects, initiating a lot of contacts and new relations, spending a lot of money, having great ideas and being creative. He started writing poems, took up singing, dancing, and many other activities. But common to them all, it seemed he never finished any of these projects. The only thing he seemed to finish was his climbing expeditions. In hindsight, we were all very happy that he did. If he hadn't, all of us would have felt terrible and perhaps our careers would have taken a different path.

3 THE UNINHIBITED SOLDIER

During my practice as a psychiatrist, I've met individuals working in the armed forces a couple of times. In view of the type of challenges they expose themselves to, it may not be obvious to all, but in fact they are like anyone else in most senses, even in terms of diseases and issues of the mind as I have observed from my profession. The type of issues that they have shown is thus just a reflection of what you will find in the general population. However, from time to time I have met individuals who have had mind issues, making it difficult for them to work and function as soldiers especially, and sometimes even making it impossible to serve in the military at all. It is not particularly surprising that most of the time it is the Post-Traumatic Stress Syndrome that brings them to the psychiatrist. But there have also been cases where the mind issues have been dropping down as from a clear blue sky with really nothing to explain why, and nothing that can be recalled that preceded it. The story about The Uninhibited Soldier is taken from one of these cases and is completely different from what you would commonly see in any normal population. The Uninhibited Soldier would turn concepts upside down and would affect everyone in his surroundings.

For Billy it all started when he was serving in the North of Sweden, in Kiruna, as a Lieutenant in the Search and Destroy Forces. Billy had been married and had two children, a daughter and a son, but he was living by himself. His wife had left him about three years earlier and had moved far away from this far-north town, all the way down to the south-west coast of Sweden, taking with her the two children for whom she had full custody. For that reason Billy seldom visited his children, and he missed them dearly. He was 45 years old and had been serving in the Armed Forces as a running soldier, being an expert on movable armoury and heavy machine guns.

For the last few years he had mainly been working as a teacher in care of the training of new recruits within the camp. Somehow he had become unfocused and was not fulfilling his duties in terms of teaching and the administrative tasks in the way he used to, and he had gotten several reminders from his boss, one of the Majors of the regiment. In spite of these "soft warnings" he seemed not to care too much about it. His colleagues were surprised by his carelessness. One of his closest friends, Lars, asked him how he was doing and why he seemed so relaxed, but Billy just answered that he felt there was nothing to worry about. This carelessness would slowly evolve, and with this style of his, he appeared more and more challenging to his colleagues – especially to his boss.

One day Billy arrived at the morning meeting untidy and not dressed according to the regulations. This was clearly too-strong of a provocation, and this time his boss had had it and gave him a warning in front of his colleagues. He also asked him to come by his office after the meeting. Perhaps this was sufficient since this time Billy remained silent for the rest of the meeting – something that was very unusual for Billy. He almost always interacted and asked questions during most meetings. He did not speak to his friends about it, but one friend, Lars, checked on him. Once more Billy seemed completely fine with the situation. This would, however, turn out not to be the last unlucky event for Billy: just a few days later he came to an official event having "forgotten his tie and being unshaved", and he was once more summoned to his boss.

A few days later as Billy was instructing a group of recruits, he told one of them to start shouting. "This is what you do when you want to get attention," said Billy to the recruit, and he began shouting to demonstrate how a proper soldier of his rank would do it. Billy was not a drill sergeant and this was not that type of exercise. It all seemed very inappropriate, and the recruit raised his voice out of respect for Billy, but not nearly as loud as Billy did, which made Billy challenge him even more. All this sudden shouting made the group anxious, and they started to look around to see if someone else had reacted to this odd scene.

It all might have passed unnoticed if it weren't for some of Billy's colleagues passing by the training area who observed this strange behaviour. As most of us know, being disciplined and in control is very important in the armed forces and inherent in their concept of the leadership. Shouting may also be common in the military, but not in an uncontrolled manner. Thus, the lack of control and discipline that Billy demonstrated as a leader – especially in front of the new recruits – was extraordinary and obviously could not be tolerated. Something had to be done immediately. Imagine if a reaction were evoked among the recruits: possible disagreements and disappointments could arise and unwanted behaviour could spread. To stop this from going viral, Billy was immediately withdrawn from active duty. His boss asked him to go home and he would later call Billy to arrange a meeting with the psychologist and physician at the camp to initiate an investigation.

The major probably thought that doing so had brought the problem under control. However, this would turn out not to be the case. Although Billy went home and stayed away from work for a while, he returned a few hours later – at 3 o'clock in the morning. The guard at the gate was unaware of the turmoil and let Billy in. Since there were no cameras at the gate, we do not know exactly what Billy did, but he left traces of his belongings (such as his jacket) in the main office where his boss worked. The next morning, there in the main office, the boss found his desk littered with cigarette butts lying among the binders and books as if Billy had attempted to study in the middle of the night at his boss' desk. The restroom was found in a bad shape with two toilets not being flushed and a dirty towel being left on the ground. When the guard made one of his regular inspections he found Billy sleeping on the floor just outside his boss' office.

Since Billy was an officer and since he seemed confused when he woke up, the guard took him to the hospital and later called the Major to report on the event. Somehow, Billy managed to escape from the hospital and went straight home to his apartment without any real investigation being undertaken. The Major, who had just arrived at his office, decided to call Billy. According to the major's report, he tried to have a serious conversation with him, but Billy seemed inattentive and confused, interrupting with vague words that his boss couldn't understand.

So what could Billy have been suffering from, and why did he speak like he had his mouth full of hot water? Could he have been under the influence of alcohol, or even drugs? Was he psychotic or in a crisis? Was he suffering from a somatic illness? At this point in time, the AIDS epidemic had just started, and many who were not at risk feared it would spread uncontrollably. There were stories about viruses affecting the brain. Could this have been Billy's case? Suddenly during the talk with his boss, Billy just left the phone on the table and the Major could hear him leave his apartment and close the door.

So what had happened then with Billy? Did he once more try to return to his work or did he spontaneously decide to do something else? It turned out that Billy went out to his car, and without much preparation began a long journey through the stretch of Sweden. Through forest and fields, from the northern landscapes heading south, he drove and drove until he thought he had reached his goal. In this state that he was in he must have been a potentially dangerous driver, but amazingly, there was only one report of an issue that came in afterwards. Usually, when you drive through Sweden from the north to the south it would take several days and you would be expected to take many breaks and stay at hotels to get some good rest before the next stretch. Perhaps it would normally take from three to five days if you drove about ten hours each day. It seemed that Billy had done this journey in just two days. He did not make it all the way through, but he was noticed at a big parking place some 300 km north-east of Gothenburg. Someone had seen a man behaving strangely walking back and forth restlessly speaking to himself. This was before the time of the mobile phones and Bluetooth headphones, so it seemed very odd indeed to see a person talking to himself like this. No one dared to approach him, but a few drivers began to discuss among themselves what to do. The man seemed disturbed in some sort of way, and action must be taken. They talked to the owner of a gas station close by, and soon the police entered the scene to make an inquiry.

This was in the summer time, and there were worries about car theft and drunken tourists at this place where so many cars stopped every day, so this probably explained the urgency that the other drivers felt. The policemen approached Billy who seemed completely confused and agitated. He walked back and forth not paying attention to their questions and not being aware that he suddenly was no longer alone. What Billy said didn't make any sense, but a few sentences or words were intelligible. The officers could clearly hear him say that he wanted to go to Gothenburg to see his daughter (among all the other gibberish he produced). After having gotten closer to Billy they were able to have him sit down in the police car. They noticed that he had no identification, but only some cash. Via the police radio and some support from the office, they used the car's license plate number to identify Billy. Since he was so confused, the police took him to a local physician, a general practitioner, who did his best in trying to examine him.

However, Billy was not in a frame of mind to let anyone examine him just like that, and he refused to cooperate. He clearly was confused, agitated, and perhaps even psychotic: he rejected normal interaction and communication. The General practitioner and the two policemen conferred, and it could not be ruled out that, with his behaviour, he may be dangerous to himself or (even worse) to someone else. Based on all of this, the physician decided to write a "statement of acute mental illness" in order to have Billy taken to a psychiatrist for further examination and treatment. And so he arrived, with the help of the police, to the psychiatric unit of the region, still some 250 kilometres from Gothenburg – the place where he wanted to be.

He stayed in this other town for a week and was investigated independently by two psychiatrists. His legal situation was confirmed. Step-by-step and with the help of anti-psychotic medication, he eventually calmed down and got some rest, enabling him to eat and drink properly, which further stabilized his health status. After a few days he was in such a good state that the nurse was able, at least in part, to have a sensible conversation with him.

Billy was still not completely coherent, and he spoke in short and concrete sentences. He said he was from the military, a soldier, and he was from the North. He was on his way to see his daughter who lived in Gothenburg. This all seemed correct since the nurse by now knew that he had repeated this information a couple of times. The nurse had to ask specific questions to pull out more information, and she learnt that he also had a son who lived in Gothenburg, although for some reason he exclusively asked about his daughter. She noticed that Billy tended to repeat some words and sentences and was overall slightly confused and restless. The psychiatric team was under the impression that Billy suffered from a psychosis, but the language disturbances together with the other findings were not fitting into any known disease entity that they were familiar with. The overall psychiatric picture was pointing in several directions, and one of the psychiatrists came to the conclusion that it must be due to an organic psychosis.

The psychiatric team sent Billy for a computerized tomography of his brain which, to their great surprise, revealed what looked like a massive atrophy in the frontal parts of the brain. They had never seen anything like this before, at least not of this magnitude, and they worried that it may be due to something that was evolving rapidly, such as encephalitis. Once again the discussion on AIDS came up, and although both psychiatrists found that possibility rather unlikely, it was kept among several hypotheses as a potential cause of the syndrome from which Billy suffered. The nurse was given instructions to draw and handle blood samples with caution.

Meanwhile, Billy spent his days walking around the department talking to other patients and speaking about his experiences as a soldier in an uninhibited way. He was told several times to stay within the limits, but he just could not help himself. It seemed that words and odd behaviours just poured out of him.

The results of the blood test came in a few days later, and all seemed to be normal, including the HIV test, thus not giving any clues as to what may have caused the atrophy. The psychiatrists conferred and decided to send Billy to the specialist clinic in Gothenburg where further investigations could be undertaken. The placement did not take long, and since Billy was still regarded as unreliable, lacking insight into his illness, and potentially harmful to himself, he was sent with the help of law enforcement to the specialist unit in the region in Gothenburg. Finally, he was about to arrive at his desired destination.

Considering the state of mind that Billy was in, it was quite surprising that he managed to drive all the way through Sweden by himself: Sweden is a geographically long country with many good roads, but it has a varying landscape that can be challenging if a driver is not fully attentive. So many things could have gone wrong, and so much could have happened on the way. He was, (considering his state of mind) potentially dangerous to other people – at least in a situation where he was behind the steering wheel of a car.

After a three-hour trip, Billy arrived in Gothenburg at the neuropsychiatric clinic where I worked at the time. He went through a number of investigations – some of his brain, some of his somatic functions, and soon it was time for all professionals involved to analyse and discuss, to go through all observations, to debate and contemplate, and to diagnose and find a suitable treatment for Billy. That meant that Billy was left to the care and observation of the staff at the neuropsychiatric ward as he waited for the results.

Passive as it may sound awaiting the results at the ward, there was a daily activity program for the patients. There was a structure which was very important to Billy, and at least he had arrived in the city where his children lived. At the same time, this was an excellent opportunity for me as the Chief Physician of the ward to continue observing him, interacting with him, and getting to know him, all of which was critical in determining the most probable diagnosis and functional level.

After lunch some patients had returned to their beds to rest and some were off to further investigations, so I had some extra time to talk to Billy. He was walking in the corridor of the ward, and if a door was open he would gaze into the room, looking like he was about to explore the premises, either by entering or perhaps just from a distance. I walked up to him and said, "Hello."

He turned around with his whole body and embraced me with a big smile which quickly wore off and turned into a more curious-looking facial expression. He did not respond to my questions but counteracted by asking when he could see his daughter. This was a fair question, and I started to present some options when he interrupted me and said, "You are the doctor, right?"

I barely had time to respond when he said, "I am not ill, you know. I have a stomach ache, but I am not ill. Is that why I am here? For my stomach ache?"

He stared at me with wide-open eyes while I asked if he wanted me to investigate his stomach. He nodded, and off we went to the physician's office. We went in silence and entered into the room where he looked around and stood by the investigation bed waiting for me to start.

There in the examination room Billy was restless and easily

distracted. He had difficulties answering my questions to the full extent: he gave short answers and then asked me what time it was, when he was going to be let out, when would it be lunch time and if I worked here at the department. Although I could only retrieve a little from the interview with him, I could capture much more by observing him. He displayed symptoms such as being easily distracted, having difficulty concentrating on a subject, being restless, repeating certain words and coming back to particular questions that he also repeated. He also showed signs of being uninhibited whenever he asked questions of his fellow patients at the ward and also of myself. He seemed to have an increased temper; he was lightly agitated while normally he was basically unemotional or of a neutral mood. He had difficulties with time orientation, but it was clear that he knew where he was and who he was, and he could also tell a little bit about what had happened over the last few days.

When I started to examine him he took the reflex hammer from me before I realized what was happening and then swung it through the air down to his knee to tap himself with it. He did not hit the muscle, but rather the knee cap, and so no reflex was released. He seemed totally absorbed by the motion and hit himself over and over. Then he stopped and looked up at me. "I am a doctor," he said with complete sincerity.

He seemed slightly on the verge of examining me, so I asked him if he was done examining himself and if he hadn't forgotten to test the plantar reflex, the Babinsky's test [11]. He looked at me with big questioning eyes, and I could read his confusion. But he found a way out and asked me to do it for him, so I went on to ask him to lie down on the couch and relax. Then I moved towards his feet and took one of them in my hand and scratched the pedal side of it

---

[11] The plantar reflex (or Babinsky's test) is a reflex elicited when the sole of the foot is stimulated with a blunt instrument.

with the shaft of the hammer. He quickly retracted his feet and looked at me, but we were fully into the examination, and it was clear we should complete it.

Positive Babinski reflexes were released on both feet implying that either he was one of the few that had this phenomenon habitually or that it was due to a lesion in his brain (which was more likely). When I asked him why he was here at the department he had no clear idea or explanation. He said that he was at the hospital and that he has pain in his knees, but he just did not seem to be able to connect the dots.

I was not at the unit that day when he finally met his daughter. I learnt about it afterwards from the staff and from Mary, his daughter, herself. It happened at the ward just a few days after he arrived. She came by and called on the entrance to the locked neuropsychiatric ward where he was staying. One of the nurses opened the door and let her in. As if Billy felt it was about to happen – as if he were clairvoyant – he rushed out of one of the rooms which he was currently exploring and kept his eyes fixed on the entrance. The two spotted each other almost simultaneously and he walked as fast as he could, almost running like a little child, towards her. She knew it was her father, but she stood completely still and opened her arms slowly as he approached her. It had been such a long time since they had been together, and the way he moved towards her was slightly odd. They stood there hugging for a few seconds. Billy then looked at her and gave her a big smile. But that was all there was to it. Whatever she had expected from him in terms of emotions he had given to her. Afterwards he was back to his repeated utterances, his almost-staccato voice, talking through her, not to her.

While he looked at her, his conversation seemed out of sync with the situation. He talked about himself. Occasionally he seemed joyful, although only briefly; the affects were quickly gone as if they were just hints or illusions. The two sat down in a meeting room, and he talked and talked. When she had listened to him for perhaps an hour or so she felt it was time to go home, but he didn't accept her leaving. He wanted her to stay and started questioning why she was going. When she said she could stay a few minutes more, he immediately continued where he had stopped. This was her first experience as a grown up with her father and she didn't know what to think. She had no reference to what he suffered from, and she felt awkward most of the time she was with him. Still, that he had driven through the stretch of Sweden just to see her was a response to her long-held longing for him, and she couldn't help feeling a bit warm inside. She saw an older version of her brother in him just in the way he looked and perhaps in his voice. But in so many ways he was different from anyone she had ever met. How could this be? Had he always been like that or had it developed after the family left? And, among the most terrifying thoughts she had ever had was this: would she become like him?

"I never got to know my father." The words came out as a statement about someone who was dead, but it was said with tenderness while she looked at me with big eyes – such eyes that only innocent teenagers may have. "I know they quarrelled a lot, and then we left, but I was too young to know who he really was." She paused, and her gaze focused on a point far away. "I have felt such a strong longing for my father, but now I don't know what to think." A trace of a tear was growing in her eye but never came out. "Now that I see him he is so strange. Whatever I remembered about him was not like this." She halted once more and looked at the examining table, then exhaled and swallowed and turned back her eyes at me.

"I clearly recall his enthusiasm for us and the joy we felt when he was playing with us – with me and my brother. We used to have so much fun when I was a child. I also recall his warm hugs when he tucked us into bed at night. Now I worry that I myself will walk the same path as he – that I will become like him." This time she could not hold back, but the tear started to run down her chin. As if time had stopped and we had frozen with it, nothing happened for a few seconds. She then wiped her eyes with the tissue that lay on the table. I did my best in meeting her in this state of mind that she was in – acknowledging the worry that she felt. Slowly, we left this zone of angst and started to talk about what it was that he was suffering from. I walked her through all the investigations made, painting the medical picture, explaining what it meant for Billy and how symptoms and signs fit with the brain changes that were observed. She asked a lot of questions and was, to my surprise, very interested in the medical and scientific part. She asked about the prognosis as merely one of several relevant questions.

Billy's ex-wife had moved as far away from him as she could ever imagine while still staying within the borders of the same country. And in spite of his illness, it had still taken a lot of convincing to get her to the Hospital for a meeting with me. She said she never wanted to talk with or about him ever again. It was overly clear she was hurt into the depth of her soul. She sighed and paused. I waited.

"This will be hard for me", she continued. They had been lovers and had built a family life together. "From my daughter I know he is ill, but to me he is still devilish". There was another pause, and the room shivered in tense silence. "He was mean to me, you know. I had to endure his mean attacks and evil tongue for two years before I found no other way out than to leave him and take the kids with me. I had witnesses, not only my two kids, who perhaps were a bit too young to fully understand, but still they saw him in action. And I had two friends who by mistake had some unpleasant experiences with his untamed and strange behaviour."

"What was it that he said to you?" I asked boldly.

"He was mean and manipulative; he said he was going to do things to help but changed his mind, leaving me in trouble." She stopped and looked away as if she was about to cry. From the look on her face, the part not turned away, she struggled to hide her tears. After a while (perhaps a minute) of silence, she turned her head back but looked down at the table when she described his manners.

"It started with a few arguments about small things. He accused me of different things which soon turned into big quarrels. I didn't understand why in the beginning and perhaps neither later on. Perhaps I still don't. At least I will never accept it. He even tried to steal my kids from me."

"Are they both your children, and is Billy the biological father?" I asked.

"Yes. What he did was to try to spread a rumour that I was bad for my kids. He told lies to our neighbours saying that I neglected them. However, they never believed him, and since we were so well-acquainted and had met at social occasions several times, they knew what he said was wrong. One of my better friends, whom he also tried to convince, told me that he said it in such a strange way. He was sort of a bad liar. After some time when I had confronted him with these lies, he began to threaten me, and he did it over and over again. It was when he started to grab me and hurt me that I knew I had to leave."

She never had to meet him again. We talked and left it there. Her input was valuable for us to better understand the progression of the disease, and it was clear that something had already happened way before he started to lose control over his work. Not surprisingly, family life may be the first indicator that something is wrong. However, acceptance, as a law of nature, is the greatest within a family, and even severe behavioural changes may be assimilated and compensated for by family members. It is not to be expected that anyone would know this. But if there were ways to detect these disorders earlier, some families would have a better chance to remain intact. But as of today, science has many steps to take before this vision may be fulfilled, at least with regard to neuropsychiatric disorders.

Instead of Billy's ex-wife, it was his teenage daughter who became his closest ally, being there for him (and perhaps for herself, too) whenever she had a chance to.

When the team started to summarize the findings from the investigations made, the most striking discovery was a severe degeneration of the frontal areas of Billy's brain. This was associated with a clearly reduced blood flow in the corresponding brain regions. All other medical investigations were normal, including an EEG. Neuropsychiatric and psychological investigations revealed clear signs of a frontal brain syndrome which, in Billy's case, was characterized by a clear change in personality, difficulties in planning and executing, a lack of inhibition so that words and acts came out without any control. In addition, there was jocularity and often an elevated mood. It matched with a diagnosis of frontotemporal dementia, possibly with an underlying Pick's disease[12].

This may or may not make any sense, and it may just represent empty or refined academic terms without any relevance to the patient, the spouse and their relatives. However, to the family it provided some explanation, especially the relationship between changes in the brain and the symptoms that occurred, although they had never before encountered this unusual disease. For Billy, on the other hand, anything done or said was irrelevant, as he more or less was living in a world of his own. And for me, as the Hippocratic Oath for physicians states, we should "sometimes cure" and "often treat" when there is no cure. All that was left to consider was to try to treat some of the most disruptive of Billy's behaviours and always comfort and arrange for good care of him. This meant that Billy had to stay a couple of weeks at the ward before proper care could be arranged.

Days passed at the ward, and it was during this period in time

---

[12] http://en.wikipedia.org/wiki/Pick's_disease

that I wanted to make an appointment with his employer. I went into the physician's office and dialled the number I had received from the nurse the day before. The phone rang a few times without an answer, and I thought at first that I may need to dial another day or even later that same day. But finally his boss answered the phone.

He had a rather tense voice at first, but he began to relax with time as we spoke about Billy. He acknowledged that they had received the notice about Billy, and they had already started to prepare for changes to accommodate for his absence from work. At first he spoke from a professional viewpoint, and it was only when I asked him how he had been personally affected that he hesitated and started to tell more in his own words about what had happened. He probably realized that I was not someone that cared about his career, but rather about people – especially Billy – and how to help him in the best way. He told me how irritated he had been for quite a while and how much extra work Billy had generated by not following instructions and agreed-upon plans and basically not doing what he used to do. It had taken him a while to realize that something may be wrong with Billy. At first he just found him annoying. But when Billy started to behave strangely, such as when he made noises and shouted without warning – when he directed the new recruits to do mad things – it just was too odd to be part of something within the normal range of behaviours. He told me he had started to dislike Billy, which he now regretted. Because he knew Billy for many years, he thought Billy had changed and perhaps was evolving into a personal catastrophe – into a devilish demon that would plague him and his colleagues for quite a while.

The explanation that I gave him was kind of a relief. We talked perhaps for an hour, and basically I just needed to kick-start him to have him continue talking without stopping for the stretch of the hour.

Over a week later, plans for Billy's care were finally decided.

A team of coordinating community officers had found the proper placement for Billy; a small nursing home for individuals with organic brain changes. It was about an hour's drive from Gothenburg. His daughter had joined in the meeting as did Billy, although he was relieved from further duty after about ten minutes of chatting about his new project, completely irrelevant to the objective of the meeting. And although he was the main attraction of the meeting, his presence distracted the other team members too much. Billy was nevertheless happy to leave the meeting: as usual, he did not really care about feedback or comments. He was in his own world and as happy as ever.

His destination was decided not by will, desire, nor ideology, but solely by biology. He was to spend a few years at a nursing home for patients with brain lesions, which by the way was named after one the local neurologists who spent many years reporting on the effects of brain lesions in various reports, articles and in books as well as delivering lectures also to the public. There Billy became somewhat of a leader for the others. The combination of his ample storytelling, everlasting enthusiasm, and wild, uninhibited ideas made it easy for others to find enjoyment in his company. For some of them, this was a change in the usual rather dull and uneventful life they spent there, and Billy became a beacon in this dark grey shadow land.

Billy enjoyed the position he earned by bringing adventure to their routine-packed days. It wasn't planned: it all just happened. On one of those dreary days, Billy came up with an idea to escape from the home. He had not thought it through, and due to their neurological disabilities it was actually impossible for most of them to be a part of such an enterprise. But there were a few that could, and although Billy didn't approach them at first (he just talked randomly to anyone close-by, so it did not come to the attention of the guards), he managed to gather a group of four comrades who, with Billy's help, managed to open the gate and flee. They had run into the forest and fortunately soon found a road which they followed. According to the others who were able to tell their version of the event, they had a lot of fun, and Billy was as entertaining as ever. Billy would never talk about it, and when asked, he started to talk about new adventures. He was always willing to share his impulsive plans with anyone.

But the disease progressed, and soon Billy became too degenerate to be able to stay at this place; a new plan was needed. By that time it had become clear within the region that there was an increasing need for nursing homes that specialized in different types of patient handicaps and behaviours. Billy would need to move back to Gothenburg into one of the recently-opened homes for severely handicapped patients.

Back then, about once a year I would take a whole day off to travel within the region to visit old patients that I had investigated before in order to learn of how they were doing. When I saw him there, being completely bedridden, unable to move arms and legs, it was beyond my imagination how that could happen to someone like Billy. I had, of course, seen many bedridden and severely degenerate patients. But it was just a few years ago that he was able to do most of what we expect from someone who is completely healthy. This was a shock to me to see him in this state, and I almost lost my breath for a few seconds. His face was also affected, torn down by the aging process, not so much with wrinkles, but more the look of a person, who was ill – dehydrated and pale. His hair was all grey in spite of him being just a little more than 50 years of age. I had met several patients with paralysis, and in Billy´s case it was due to a loss of motor neurons in the spine, but still I wasn't fully prepared for this.

Billy, on the other hand, was as ready as ever. When I entered his room, a white-grey, clean and meagre hospital-type of bedroom, he instantly gave me a big smile shining with everything he had. My conflicting feelings gave way to his obvious cheerfulness, and I walked towards him with my hand stretched out. He could, of course, not respond but I saw him trembling with joy. I stayed there just watching him, talking to him and telling how happy I was to see him. In spite of all the gloominess of the hospital environment, in spite of his severe state, it was a happy moment for both of us.

This was the last time I saw Billy. He died less than a year after my visit, and all that was left was a lot of memories and a few biological samples donated to research. From these it was later concluded that Billy had suffered a motor neuron disease with severe affection of the frontal lobes[13].

---

[13] Bak. Ann Indian Acad Neurol. Dec 2010; 13(Suppl2): S81–S88.

4 SPEED TO OVERCOME MOVEMENT

This is the story of a young man called John who entered into his twenties with a smile on his face knowing that he carried the gene for Huntington's disease. He had inherited it from his father who was long-since gone. His nervous system was being torn apart while he, with all his courage and will power, chose to look the other direction. And what he found there, being it friends, love, good times and joy, was what kept him going. For as long as anyone knew, he remained on top of and mastered the forces that inevitably, like a law of nature, would bring him down. In every sense there is, he was a remarkable and admirable young man.

It was told that John's father had died in a car accident when John was merely one year old, and the boy basically grew up under the care of his mother. His childhood was normal, and he went through preschool and grade school being just like any other kid: learning, playing, running and fooling around. He had his first love affair, his first success as an athlete and his first fight as a young teenager. He was a natural in sports and was popular, swiftly gaining a large network of friends. School was a social environment, and he thrived from being around so many people. Still, he did not know about his inheritance, since his mother had decided to spare him the message until he had passed the fiercest period of adolescence. It was when he was about 17 that she took him for a long journey through Sweden, stopping by at a rented cottage in the beautiful highlands of Dalarna, where she was certain they would be alone and have the time to go through it all.

They experienced two weeks of hell together. John's reaction was that of a crisis, and he went from the mechanical behaviours of shock to the outburst of a severe reaction, which turned out to be both a mental and physical struggle. Leaving the cottage, he was in a state of depression as he slowly started to assimilate the facts.

After he got home, his friends soon found out. They reacted as true friends do and walked the path with him to his recovery from the melancholia. It was then that he made some of the most important decisions of his life, and his life would change in so many ways.

When I met him several years later, his choreatic movements were already established, and he had severe difficulty in moving. He had to be helped with eating and getting dressed and supported when attempting to walk. But the real problem which lay behind so many of his visits to the ward were the frequent periods of heavy drinking and abuse of narcotic medication. While no one really could blame him, and while it was difficult to influence the different mechanisms that acted to maintain this pattern, it still was a problem for him and everyone around him.

Every time he was drunk it especially affected everyone around him since he shouted and acted in an uninhibited manner and could become quite angry. This would also make it more difficult for others to help him, and sometimes he even lost control of his bladder and bowels, which was disturbing to all and an embarrassment to him. During these periods it quickly became too intense and heavy for them all, and thus treatment and care at the hospital was necessary.

John was sitting in a corridor in a wheelchair looking quite drowsy and apathetic while his movements were jerky and myoclonic as ever. I approached him and started to talk to him, wanting to know how he felt, but he just briefly looked at me and then continued to stare into the long corridor in which he was sitting. I tried a few more times, but there was no way that I could get his attention. His mother had just arrived, so I decided to talk to her instead.

We sat down in my office and she immediately was quite frank and told me what had happened and why he was there. She apologized that this had happened so many times. She also confessed that it was just too difficult not to let him be happy (as he was when he started to drink). She told me of the intense and overflowing pain she felt when he was suffering and the relief she felt when he started to relax and then get excited after a few drinks. She then cried, a soft, almost quiet cry, with tears running down her cheeks. The conversation stopped and she looked at me with eyes all wet. So we sat there together, letting the sadness pass.

The next day, John's mother arrived early and approached me to continue her story. Obviously, she felt stronger today and had decided to give me more background. I recall we swiftly got into the heart of the matter. She told me that when John went into one of his drinking periods, he usually would behave strangely for a time after he stopped drinking, as if he were paranoid: he avoided talking. She thought this was due to a combination of exhaustion and bluntness, which was not only a sign of abstinence but also an evolving sign of personality change that followed as the disease progressed. Even when he was not abstinent he could sometimes behave in this manner, but it was especially common after a period of drinking. It would usually take him at least a week to recover from alcohol intake. With this information, I decided to give him some time to recover, which meant it would be a few days before I approached him again to have a conversation with him.

John had been at the department for several episodes during the last few years, and he was well known to the staff. Several of the staff had also worked there for many years and had spent a lot of time with him, taking him out for walks in a wheelchair or sometimes to a cafe close-by. John was well-liked among the staff, and his uncontrolled movements along with his occasional wittiness led to a lot of empathy and liking among the staff and his friends. His symptoms were as severe as ever, and in spite of the neurologist having tried to help him with various medications, there seemed to be nothing that really could stop the movements.

As with all patients with Huntington's disease, it's emotionally heart breaking to watch them try to move while being as affected as they are by all the involuntary movements. The intense and very sudden myoclonic[14] jerks, the ballistic form of almost explosive movement of arms and legs and the grimacing that never seems to stop make it ever so difficult to interpret how they are and how they feel. Although you may get a better impression when you talk to them, there are still so many things that affect their ability to communicate verbally and express what they feel. It's basically only when looking at their eyes that you can tell whether they are alert, drowsy, sad or at least okay.

It was about a week after he arrived at the department that we finally sat down to talk again. He then told me that he felt better and that he had started to sleep more during the nights. He was regretful that he had been drinking alcohol, but at the same time he told me that it gave him much pleasure and joy. Without my asking him, he then told me how much he liked drinking alcohol and how important that had become in his life. When he was young, before the onset of the disease, alcohol was nothing more than a symbol of protest of the adult world and doing what was prohibited. In the same way drugs were just a way of challenging the expectations and the rules. He was drunk a couple of times as a kid, but it really wasn't until the onset of his disease and when the neurological symptoms and signs started to create boundaries for him that drinking came to provide him with something that he since praised. It was a solace, a relief and a joy. He enjoyed the happiness he felt when the effects of alcohol started to kick in, relaxing his muscle tone, exciting his senses and soothing his overcharged brain. It was almost as if he had found the cure that he had been looking for as a young adult, and every time he was drunk, it brought him close to what he felt was at least borderline-to-normal.

Of course, there were the side effects, like the headache and the day-after nausea and tiredness. But his addiction and the craving were immediate and complete for him, all due to the very positive

---

[14] a brief, involuntary twitching of a **muscle** or a group of muscles.

experiences he had from the state of excitement while being drunk. It was all that he wanted. Beginning with the first signs of arousal and excitement as the alcohol effects started to kick in, then moving after perhaps an hour into a state of relaxation that he could maintain for several hours, it brought him so much pleasure and relief that it was as close to a complete solution or a cure as he thought he could come.

As the disease progressed and his symptoms and signs became worse and more severe, the longing and craving for alcohol increased. He knew the aftermath was a pain both to him and especially to his mother, but that was in no way nearly as bad as the disease itself, and not even close to stopping him from doing it again. He had told his mother at an early stage of his disease that this was important to him, and she accepted it. She had always wanted the best for him, and even with this toxic, this chronic poisoning, she could see with her own eyes how happy he was when he drank. And so it became important also to her that he could maintain this habit.

John went on to speak about how he had decided to live his life. He had made this decision a long time ago almost as far back as he could remember. He thought he must have been a small child when he felt there was something special about him, and although there was so little information about his father while he was growing up, and though he wasn't fully aware that he also was going to be ill, he sensed that his mother and her friends took extraordinarily good care of him. In some ways he was treated differently from other children. Not that he felt spoiled or overprotected, but he felt it was important to the people around him that he feel good about himself and that he enjoy life.

Finding out one day that he carried the genes for Huntington's disease kicked off some major changes within John. Like most other people who know they are going to suffer, who know something about their future, he decided to find a cure for himself and to become an expert on the disease. He read all the information available and talked to experts, but without any relief. All that consumption of information and the fight, the struggle for and the search for something that could help him substantially to avoid the pain, eventually exhausted him. One day it just became too much for him. He literally hit the wall at one hundred kilometres per hour and fell to the ground, but without any answers and with no remedy.

After that, spending a couple of months in a state of depression, he took himself back, step-by-step (of course with the support from his mother and friends) and eventually he came to accept that he was going to live with, but never approve of, what was going to happen to him. The acceptance in itself led to other changes within him that made him to decide that he would live his life to the fullest extent for as long as he could. He would not refuse any pleasure that was presented to him, but he would take it on with every bit of his remaining vigour, energy and enthusiasm. It became the ambition, the target in his life, almost as an obsession to live life to the fullest extent. It was of utmost importance that he could feel as much freedom as possible with the little time he had left.

He, a male Cinderella without the happy finale, having a clock counting down to the inevitable end, became a party man. Every day was an opportunity to have a ball. Ever since his teenage days, he was the first to try everything: girls, alcohol, drugs, illegal acts, dangerous missions, pushing the limits and seizing the day as much and as often as possible.

During the time that John was at the department, there was an article in the scientific journal *Nature*[15] about a potential future treatment to reduce the signs of Huntington's disease. In an animal disease model of Huntington's disease, one of the most common antibiotics was tried and turned out to silence the disease-

---

[15] *Nature Medicine* **6**, 797 - 801 (2000) doi:10.1038/77528

generating genes, thereby in a sense temporarily curing the disease. This was great news, especially since the treatment was already available for humans. However, there were many unanswered questions such as:
- Would the drug work at all in patients?
- If so, at what dose?
- What additional risks it would carry for long term treatment?

Still, a glimmer of hope was lit in me, and I decided to present the idea of treating patients to some of my colleagues that were specialists in neuropsychiatry and neurology. To my great surprise, I was met almost exclusively with a lot of scepticism. Even though it put me off for a few hours, I decided not to give up; I called the medical research council to discuss what was needed to get a license to try this treatment. Even there I was met with some scepticism and concern, especially since the study was done in animals and thus, it may not work in humans, furtheremore about the presumably high doses and the extended duration of time that the treatment needed to have an effect. I was asked if I was prepared to take the risk. This time, I felt less convinced, and so I put the idea on the shelf for a few days to give me some time to reflect and digest all the disturbing feedback.

A week went by, and then I was ready to give it another chance. I called one of the leading experts in Sweden to discuss whether this was something that he would try himself. This time, fortunately, I was finally met with the same type of enthusiasm that I myself felt. But after a long conversation (perhaps had it been an hour), after we had discussed mechanisms, doses, where the effects would be visible, and the possible side-effects and risks, the conversation took a sudden turn, and he said, after pausing for a few seconds, that he still felt that the risks with prolonged treatment at such doses was not something that he could recommend. Instead he gave me specific advice on currently available treatments that at least would provide some relief for

John. He thanked me for a "wonderful and exciting" discussion and encouraged me to follow up soon. Then we ended the call, and I sat still, staring out into the empty space in front of me as if I had lost my vision, feeling very clearly that this was the last bullet that I had. My contemplation and impression of all this "risk averseness" finally took over and dampened my initial enthusiasm. It took me, however, a few days to get over it, and I didn't feel like doing any of the other scientific tasks that I had going on at the time. With a saddened mind, I decided not to try the treatment on John. In fact, I never brought the subject to his attention or to anyone else in his surroundings.

Instead I consulted our neurologist and we initiated treatment with Tetrabenazine, the symptomatic relief approved for Huntington's disease. I instructed the nurse and informed John and his mother about the treatment, and there was no objection or concerns. Shortly afterwards, we started. There was nothing more to it, really. No one expected any revolutionary effect – especially not I – but I felt strongly that keeping my professionalism was essential as was my attempt to try to find something really helpful for John. I don't think John or his mother expected any great effects either, but he was willing to try what was available.

After perhaps a week or two, there was hardly any effect, but after that initial period we could see some slight decrease in his motor symptoms. This change, although small, seemed to make a difference to John. He told us he felt slightly better and could control his movements a little more. Now, it seemed, he was getting ready to go home, so we prepared for a release meeting. However, it turned out that we still weren't there: we had some more work to do.

One morning, perhaps two weeks after we started the Tetrabenazine treatment, I arrived as usual at the department at about eight-thirty and walked in to the nurses' office where a morning meeting was being held. The nurse on call stopped the reporting and said to me, "John has been crying all night. Nothing has been able to soothe his sorrow."

This was a surprising and sudden change that needed immediate attention. It could be a sign of anything from a psychological reaction, pain, anxiety or side effects of the medication to a whole range of other things that he was exposed to. A thorough investigation was needed. I went straight into his room and noticed the remarkable change in John. If it weren't for his disorder, you could say, beyond any reason, that he was sad. But it had all appeared so suddenly, basically from one day to the next. I did a thorough investigation on John, and we took some blood samples to rule out infection and any organ affection. We knew that Tetrabenazine could give rise to side effects, and this was the only new medication he had received in the past four weeks. I called the neurologist to get his advice.

Since the symptoms were so pronounced, we decided to drop Tetrabenazine and replace it with an antidepressant. It took about another week before the crying stopped. In fact you could say that Tetrabenazine, at least in this case and in spite of its initial positive effect, prolonged his stay at the department by several weeks. But all in all, it led to the fact that I got to know John a bit better and learned something else about him and his disorder that I found quite remarkable.

On one occasion (I cannot really recall when it was) I talked to a couple of John's friends who often visited him at the department. Several of his friends visited him, but this was a group of more frequent visitors. They were three that had been hanging around almost all that particular week, and I started to talk to them just by coincidence as they were passing by in the corridor. It started out as a nice, friendly chat, but after a while I decided to ask them if they would agree to let me interview them about John. We sat down in my office and talked for almost an hour about him.

They told me that they had been friends since early in their life, long before any of them (not even John himself) knew that he carried the gene for Huntington's disease. Thus, they had seen all the changes that John went through, all the way from the happy and playful childhood, through puberty to adulthood, and to the crisis that then hit John as the signs emerged. They went through it all and suffered with him, supported him and carried him through all of these phases – deepening their friendship as every day passed – becoming friends for life, sharing pleasure and pain, adventure and disasters. They felt they knew everything about John. They told me a lot about him, but there was particularly one thing that stayed in my mind: he was keen on high velocity, especially speed driving. He actually had a driver's license, but he had never had the time or fortune to prune his skills before the disorder took over, making it impossible for him to drive.

John spent some money on renting fast cars and talking about how much he really wanted to buy a Ferrari or a Lamborghini, but as it was with his economy, he could never afford it. Instead, his friends took him out for rides, and every time they were out they noticed how he kept on requesting that they should drive as fast as they could, whether on the motor way or a remote highway. He demanded to sit in the front seat next to the driver: John seemed to feel very much at ease with himself as the speed increased.

In the beginning, John's friends did not notice a change in him. It wasn't really that strange since, when you sit in a car which moves at a high speed, you usually look forward, even if you're not driving the car. Thus, the speed got to them all and took away the attention from what was happening with John. But it was this constant craving, this constant demanding and repeated requests from John, that made them actually start looking at him to see how he was doing during the ride. What they noticed surprised them all.

It looked like he moved less and that his jerkiness decreased as he sat there with his eyes fixed on the road that was rushing towards him. And not only so, but the more they looked at him, it seemed as if his movements diminished proportionately to the speed that the car was going. I was astonished by this tale: I had never heard anything even remotely similar. If this was true, it could provide a new opening to an understanding of what regulates body motions. So I decided that I really wanted to see it for myself.

It turned out (for several reasons) that the circumstances would not allow me to go along with him to observe this. But it was one of the staff, a young enthusiastic male, and an observant person that John trusted that had the opportunity to go with him in the car and report back to us. And indeed he came back confirming what I had heard from John's friends.

John seemed to have been totally absorbed in the speed – as if he had been pulled into it –staring with eyes fixed on the road that came running towards him with increasing speed. It was as if he was hypnotized and his presence fused with all the sights that he received from the road as it rushed towards him. This had a clear effect on decreasing his neurological movements. I talked to John about it, and he told me that this experience of everything coming towards him excited him and made him mentally forget his movements difficulties. He felt excellent when the speed increased, and longed for this experience every day. Except for alcohol it was better than anything else he had tried.

Alcohol and speed brought John to his peak. It was during these experiences that he was at his prime, and in the world of sorrow, devastation and ever-increasing, handicapping, ballistic movements, there was this thing that gave him joy and pleasure.

This all happened during the time when computer games were far from realistic. If it had been today, perhaps we could have created a virtual environment for John that would have allowed him to get into this experience as often as he liked. But back then, it was only when his friends had the time to take him out that he could enjoy the pleasures of the high speed. I have searched for an explanation of this phenomenon in the medical literature and failed to find any. Perhaps this was something unique to John, or perhaps it could help others with the same disorder. It might be that the explanation lies in a combination of arousal and brain excitement with all the visual information that is involuntarily fed into the visual centres of the brain and then spread to other parts, providing an inhibition of the neurological over activity characteristic of Huntington's disease. Whatever it was, it gave John something to look forward to.

I did not meet John for several months after that visit, and the second time I saw him was during a brief visit to the department that lasted only a couple of days. He had progressed, and his neurological signs were severely handicapping. He did not like to stay at the department then, but we made a quick adjustment to his medication, in consultation with a neurologist, in order to help him go back home as soon as possible. After that, I never saw him again during the time that I worked at that particular hospital as later I was offered a position at another hospital and moved on in my career.

I have met a few patients with Huntington's disease after this episode, although no one has told of or had the same experience as John. Obviously everyone is unique, and this improvement by experiencing the streets rushing towards him may have been exclusive to John. His faith and personality struck me in particular and the tales of him (in combination with my own despair of not being able to provide a better treatment for him) made the story stay in my memory.

In many situations nowadays, high speed and increased tempo is regarded as negative and often associated with stress. We are supposed to take it easy; we should slow down. Obviously, everyone has their own preference, and it may also be that we as scientists have more to do to explore the effects of increased speed on health. Could there be more patients such as John who may benefit from it?

5 TWENTY YEARS OF SILENCE

In today's society there seems to be less and less room for silence. We are more or less constantly surrounded by some level of noise that accompanies our presence. We usually accommodate for this, filtering out the noise and becoming completely unaware of its existence. But sometimes we notice it, letting it just pass or occasionally becoming disturbed by it. We may even get so used to it that we react by entering into periods of silence.

We may also like the noise, even crave it. Having the radio on, streaming video to the TV at the same time, having air conditioning and other electric systems keeping our internal environment in balance, having cars passing by outside our house, and talking to someone on the phone at the same time is a typical situation nowadays.

You may sometimes long for, as I do, the silence of an arctic landscape or the disciplined silence of a library or an empty meeting room. The tranquillity, the seemingly never-ending calmness in that chamber of contained air, as in contrast to the ever-present noise of the streets, may well make you feel stunned, almost weightless. But there is a balance to everything – a limit that, when crossed, turns established concepts upside down, making pleasant become bad. The story that I am about to tell you is about Tora. Silence was for her a fate, but for others it was a frustration.

For a short time in my career I worked in a small psychiatric unit located on the southwest coast of Sweden. Visitors are often struck by the charm of the pretty town and its surroundings, and every summer the population increases, and its beautiful beach is jammed with sunbathing, swimming and playing families. The landscape is full of inviting green hills and soft meadows, cottages and farms, and hardwood groves. The people in this parish are typically friendly and relaxed but prefer to keep to themselves, not interacting too much with visitors.

The history of the Psychiatric Unit of the area is remarkable in itself since it had its share of fame during the 1980's when a charismatic psychiatrist and leader, Dr Berggren, turned established concepts and rooted principles upside down. He encouraged the staff to create an inspiring atmosphere with modern and brave ideas. He reformed the psychiatric care, putting a lot of emphasis on integrity, health and freedom of the patients.

But many things had changed since then, and when I stepped in as a physician in training, which today is more than 25 years ago, only fragments of that era was left and the passion had been replaced by the so-common political tensions between different psychiatric professions.

I spent my hours mostly interviewing and investigating the in-patients, learning a lot of psychiatry and becoming especially interested in how brain lesions influence human behavioural expressions and functions. Many patients that I met made strong impressions on me, and some stories have stayed in my memory ever since. It was also here that I gained my first experiences with how various medicines impacted an individual, sometimes for better and sometimes for worse. We had medically-defendable, quality-assured rationales for all we did in the unit, but sometimes the clinical picture became clearer as time went by: explanations were mostly available in hindsight. In some cases the situation turned out well without us having a proper explanation as to why. The case I am about to relate to you is from this time and exemplifies how difficult it sometimes was (and still is) to make a clear diagnosis in spite of all scientific and medical advancements made.

Tora was about 60 years old when I met her and had spent the better part of her life in mental and psychiatric units. It should not have been like that, and no one was to be blamed for it, but whatever the reason, fate or negligence, institutional living had become her life. She grew up in the countryside a couple of miles outside of a small town and started her career at a minuscule-sized countryside school. Most of her friends were not that interested in school work, and what mattered most was what you did after school or during the breaks. But Tora was different. She was an excellent student, had high grades and was loved by her teachers and comrades. She loved to walk in the forest searching for unusual flowers and plants: biology was clearly her favourite topic.

At the age of thirteen, Tora had her first crush. He was slightly older and taller than she was and of the Bohemian type. The two of them shared the interest of spending time outdoors and had an intense love affair for a couple of weeks. They seemed to fit nicely together, but for some reason his interest diminished, and in spite of her ambitions she noticed they were fading apart. Their relationship ended when he told her had become interested in another girl.

After that, Tora had a few brief affairs or flirts during the coming years, but no lasting relationships. She graduated from high school at the age of 18 and went with her parents in their family car on vacation throughout Europe. It was during this trip that everything went completely and painfully wrong.

It happened during the night when the family had driven that extra mile on the Autobahn to reach a hotel. They did not want to stop earlier since they had already made a reservation. Rain poured down as if the sky had opened up completely, and it was dark with understandably poor visibility as if all signs were gone and no light helped to guide them. Nothing could have prevented the inevitable from happening: another car lost control and ran straight into Tora's car with high speed and unmanageable force. Like a spearhead, the car ran straight into Tora's parents. The accident ended the life of both of them as well as that of the driver of the approaching car, leaving Tora (as by a miracle) as the sole survivor with no visible injuries. She was taken to a hospital close by and investigated with all available and relevant methods, but there were no signs of any damage to her body or brain. The situation at the hospital was an atrocious experience for Tora. She did not speak German and she was described as paralyzed by fear and shaking with anxiety. The staff tried to speak English to her but she did not respond, and no one there knew how to speak Swedish. It took a couple of hours before they could locate an interpreter, but even that did not help to open her up.

Soon Tora had gone into a phase of total insulation and was staring into an empty space in front of her. Her neurological reflexes were normal and were awake, but she simply did not respond to any form of communication, especially verbal. She had to stay at the hospital a couple of days before a transfer to a psychiatric unit in Sweden could be done.

After arriving at the psychiatric unit, Tora's silence continued. During the months to come distant relatives, school friends and her former high school teacher paid her visits, talked to her, gave her hugs, and sat in silence for hours with her, but no one was able to break her seclusion. Tora displayed no signs of emotional reactions and just continued to stare into the empty space in front of her.

Tora was to stay there in the general psychiatric unit for a longer time and she had her own room. Several investigations were undertaken by different psychiatric and neurological professionals. Her language skills as well as her auditory, visual, and neurological functions were all scrutinized in depth. She underwent thorough investigations by psychologists trained in different schools using different forms of therapy, and she even underwent psychoanalytic diagnosis. The interpretations by the psychotherapists, the psychoanalyst, and therapists of all other kinds went through her life from every possible angle from birth up to the present. Among the suggested explanations for this long-lasting silence were:

- The sudden separation from her parents (This, in itself, was sufficient to induce a major grieving reaction or melancholy in Tora.)
- The accident that led to severe post-traumatic stress syndrome
- That she had suffered a brain lesion to Broca's area (the speech-generating centre of the brain)
- The guilt of surviving her parents and perhaps that she, as the only child, should have taken better care of them (trying to prevent them from going abroad) and perhaps even that she should have followed along in death
- A severe and complete psychological regression to avoid the pain of the loss of her parents

Several therapeutic approaches were consequently proposed and many tried; she had to go through them all before they were ruled out. It was, after all, a state-of-the art psychiatric unit where all therapists were regarded as equal and no therapy was superior to another. In a case such as this when it was so completely unclear what it was that caused this long-lasting muteness, it was logical that everything had to be tried.

Tora's silence in itself evoked anxiety among those who worked with her. She was a young, beautiful, talented girl who had so much of her life in front of her. With no physical injuries, she could (and should) be able to enjoy life after the grieving, but she was completely unresponsive to all that was done to her and for her.

And so time went by, months after months, years after years, and one-by-one all therapists eventually gave up their attempts at trying to get Tora to speak. Some stayed on her case for years while other left after just a few weeks. Some even took their anger out on her in despair. But still nothing happened. She was as silent as ever before. There was no reaction no matter what was tried; nothing could ever evoke a response from her. She just sat there staring in front of her doing nothing – not responding.

After some time, Tora moved into long-term care and spent time with other patients that suffered chronic psychiatric illnesses. That could have been the end of this story. She would have been placed there in a ward far away from any contact with the outside world, far away from any hope of salvation. She would just have continued to gaze into the emptiness in front of her, letting time pass slowly, waiting for her system to shut down. However, as it would prove to all who have patience, this story would turn out slightly different.

Tora's inner world began to regain its powers. With tiny bits of almost unnoticeable steps, she successively recaptured some motor functions and a slight level of independence. Some of what we regard as normal daily routines re-emerged, and some normal behaviour even came back with time, but ever so slowly. After several years, she was back to following instructions such as getting out of bed, helping in getting dressed, eating and going to the bathroom, although in all these situations she always required some assistance to complete what she was doing. After several more years, she walked around by herself. She began to brush her teeth by herself after an additional number of years, and then she began taking care of more and more of her own personal hygiene. Then she began feeding herself. But overall and from a psychiatric point of view she hadn't changed, and she was still passive, sitting quietly most of the day. Occasionally she would follow along when someone suggested they take a walk in the corridor or in the backyard, but she did not speak, and her eye contact was absent. She just seemed to be staring right through people who stood in front of her.

Although she still had not said a single word in many years and did not communicate in any other form, comparing her status from that point in time to the beginning of the silence clearly showed that she was not as frozen as she once was – at least not in motor areas. All who had the endurance to follow her would have noticed the changes. But very few, if any, had the patience. And so she was left in the care of the nursing home staff and to the belief that she was still the same: silent and still. The staff took care of her and treated her in the best way they could with love and respect.

One evening about 20 years after the accident (Tora was close to 40 years of age, it was summertime with birds singing outside, and a soft, warm breeze was shaking the leaves of the trees), something amazing happened. That evening, the patients were sitting almost randomly scattered in the main living room, and the glass doors to the garden were open to let in some hopefully cool and soothing air. Tora was, as usual, sitting in the department hall with most other patients that were unable to walk by themselves or were handicapped in other ways. Suddenly, she rose up from her chair, looked around, and started to walk to her room. (There were few staff members around, so the story is as told by the most lucent patients and by the staff.) None of the staff noticed the event until someone checked on the patients in the hall and found that she was missing. They looked around in the living room and in the hallway, but they could not find her. The first reaction was that something had happened to her. Perhaps she had fallen or been hit by another patient. This happened from time to time, but it was usually resolved quite easily. It had also happened to Tora, but only once, and it had turned out that it was an accident, an unintentional slap from a passing patient. The other patients thought she was a bit scary and usually avoided touching her.

And so they looked all around and could not find her until someone looked in her bedroom. There she was, standing in front of her bed looking unusually focused and active, packing her stuff, which by that time wasn't much, preparing to leave. She took from the drawer her blouse, a shirt and her personal hygiene tools and set them on the bed. Her movements were slow but decisive. When the staff asked her what she was doing, she responded, "I am going home". At this moment in time it was summer when a lot of the regular staff was on vacation. It was also evening, so the staff consisted of two undergraduate caretakers and a nurse who was serving several departments and was far away in the building complex. The two caretakers were stunned –flabbergasted. One of the two, Mrs Larsson, had worked for several years with Tora, and she could not believe her eyes! Now it was their time to be silent!

They stood there just watching her with amazement, not being able themselves to say a word. After a time of quietness (no one knows for how long), Mrs Larsson asked Tora, "What are you doing?"

Tora did not respond, as usual. She did mutter something as if to herself, but the words were unidentifiable. It was as if everything fell into place for her at once.

Mrs Larsson then said, "Tora, we will do anything to help you with whatever you are doing."

Tora just responded, "I am going home," then she continued to pack her belongings. She stopped only to walk around the bed in the search of things dropped on the floor.

Mrs Larsson and her colleague were so excited that they ran back to the office to call the nurse and later also physician on duty. They were going to tell night staff, the day staff, yes everyone about Tora´s remarkable change. They were going to help her home immediately. Nothing would stop them from letting Tora go home now. She was well now. The paralysis was gone and she had started to speak again. A few minutes of excitement and running back and forth in the corridor ensued with the nurse on call coming by to see what had happened. But how was it even possible? There had been no warning signals. Nothing that anyone could recall or picture had preceded this sudden and radical change. The exhilaration was total.

But as it so often is, nothing lasts forever, and luck is usually brief – a onetime event. And so it was with Tora. After having packed her stuff and combed her hair, after having told the staff she was leaving, then walking around her bed and preparing to leave, she suddenly sat down on the bed and stopped all activities.

This happened so unexpectedly and quickly that the staff had no time to react until it was too late. Her eyes slowly went back to the empty gaze she had been having for so many years. Any sparkle of life, any sign of a light in her eyes was once again gone. Any remaining movement was solely among the staff.

The next morning the staff reported on the event at the morning meeting. At first the others thought they were joking. Then they suggested they, the evening staff, were on drugs? Or perhaps they fell asleep during the watch or maybe they were simply not there at all? It was hard to imagine that something like this could have happened, but three staff members, including the nurse, were backing the story. It was also noted in the medical records. Many passed by the department that day to catch a glimpse of Tora who, just like always, was sitting still in an armchair in the main living room gazing out into an empty space in front of her. Some investigations were made once again, but there were no obvious changes as compared to before. Physically she was normal but behaviourally she was absent. She showed no response – not a single reaction – but she was completely back into the world of her own.

So what could be the explanation for this peculiar and sudden, but brief, change in this apparently chronically-ill, unendingly-suffering, and for more than 20 years mute individual? Could we find something in the theories of all the experts that many years before had tried to solve the mystery behind her silence, that suddenly, but briefly, ended? Was it indeed a psychological trauma that for so many years had put her in this state of mental paralysis? Or, could it have been the guilt of surviving when all others had died – a self-reproach that plagued her and made her chronically incompetent to start a grown-up life? Was it a personality change as in a severe regression back to early childhood, to a mentally primitive form of life? Or was it, as the neurologist proposed, a lesion to the brain area responsible for generating speech, the

Broca's area[16] and perhaps also in the RAS system[17] that made her lose her motivation and capacity to speak? Was she, perhaps, chronically melancholic?

Many professionals had been involved in trying to understand, interpret, diagnose and also treat Tora's symptoms. What was clear was that the most prevailing sign was silence, or mutism. Mutism is not as infrequent as one might imagine; however, the long duration of muteness that Tora had must be regarded as uncommon. The most common form of mutism is called "selective mutism" and is described as someone who is normally capable of speaking but who does not speak in given situations or to specific people. The frequency of selective mutism has been estimated to be one per thousand individuals; although a large study done in 2002 in Los Angeles[18] found it to be seven per thousand individuals. Selective mutism has been linked to social phobia and anxiety. However chronic mutism together with the lack of other signs or attempts from Tora to try to communicate with others should imply that there's more behind the muteness than just an anxiety disorder. In her case, it was triggered by a single, severe psychological trauma, since there was no evidence of physical damages. For that reason it is easy to exclude child development disorders such autism, in which selective and complete mutism can be found.

It could have been that mutism was caused by a brain lesion which, in some instances, may be undetectable even by Magnetic Resonance Imaging (MRI). If it had been a brain lesion, it should have been localized within the frontal lobe or in the circuitry that connects the frontal cortical areas with the more central part of the

---

[16] http://en.wikipedia.org/wiki/Broca's_area

[17] http://en.wikipedia.org/wiki/Reticular_activating_system

[18] Bergman RL, et al., J Am Acad Child Adolesc Psychiatry. 2002 Aug;41(8):938-46.

brain. It is especially the so-called Broca´s area that is known for harbouring the neuronal substrate responsible for generating language.

We don't know very much about Tora's childhood. It may have been that she, in spite of the records of her good performance in school and her excellent social capability, actually was already suffering from an evolving brain disorder such as schizophrenia. But there were no records of that, no signs described, and no reports from her friends, her relatives or her teacher that indicated that something would have been wrong before the accident.

One may speculate that a combination of a diffuse brain lesion and the psychological trauma together were strong enough factors to initiate and maintain the muteness. It is also possible that a disorder was in the development and was boosted or kicked off by this severe trauma. For instance, in schizophrenia there is a state called catatonia[19] in which mutism may occur. Mutism is often associated or combined with other symptoms and signs typical of catatonia: motor immobility and waxy flexibility of limbs, speech disturbances such as echolalia (which is mimicking what others are saying), peculiar postures and stereotyped movements. None of these were found in the case of Tora. Some physicians speculated on schizophrenia and catatonia, but a clear diagnosis was never set except for mutism. If so, treatment with ECT could have been tried, and in fact it was tried when they thought she was suffering from severe melancholia. Unfortunately, the ECT had no clear effect on her symptoms.

So why did Tora then "wake up" from this long period of silence? Was it that some kind of internal psychological or biological blockade just left for a few minutes… or was it something else? Had it happened before? Maybe this was just one

---

[19] a state of neurogenic motor immobility and behavioral abnormality manifested by stupor.

of the several or many times that Tora had "awakened", but no one had noticed it before. Our attention tends to diminish when something remains in the same state for a long period of time (that is, we sort of "de-select" it from our attention span), and it is very common to build up barriers to changes, thereby making it very difficult to notice them when they actually occur.

Now was this also the case for Tora? Had we missed this in the past, and was it now just a lucky coincidence that someone actually for once took time to notice it? But if this was just a one-time event, and the internal lock somehow was unleashed, why did she revert to becoming padlocked once more? The fact that it was recorded, mentioned and discussed did not lead to a plethora of new initiatives and new investigations. Tora was now past 40 and had been "gone" for such a long time that there were few who believed that she really could come back. Also many were sceptical of the fact that it really had happened at all (that Tora actually woke up).

The Physician responsible did a routine neurological examination and sent her for an EEG, but since both of these investigations were unable to reveal any changes in Tora, let alone any clues as to what may have happened, everything went back to the normal routine. Thus, Tora was taken care of by the nursing home, and nothing else in terms of therapeutic interventions was undertaken. Tora was once again left to herself and her state of mind.

For me, this was a temporary assignment, and I left the Psychiatric Unit after the summer never to return. Although I have met several physicians and some of the unit staff since that time, there were no real updates and no further explanations as to what really had happened to Tora. She was over 60 when I worked there and had by then been silent for more than 40 years. According to medical expertise and experience, there would be little hope that Tora would ever return to normal. It was said, "Forty years is simply too long of a time for any human to change."

6 THE ROBBING POLICE

I believe that, to many people, the men and women of the police force, along with the combination of the law enforcement, the perceived solidarity, the determination, and the selectiveness in the physical execution of their tasks, represent something archetypal in our society and thereby will be ever-fascinating to us as humans. Most often they are heroes, and what they are required to do is often extraordinary. Sometimes they are just present, conventional, and even sort of bleak. We have learnt that they, on occasion, may even cross the line and become villains.

As a psychiatrist, I have worked together with the police force in various situations, especially in emergency psychiatry. As professionals we often deal with the same societal issues, although from different viewpoints and with different objectives, but both try to help the very same individuals avoid getting lost in this complex human meshwork called "civilization".

I have also had officers in treatment, and they are, obviously, just like anyone else: they have all kinds of personal and family issues, and they represent every kind of personality that you may find elsewhere. This story that I am about to tell is about one of the more difficult cases I have had since the brain disorder that this person suffered from had consequences that affected so many people. It is the story of The Robbing Police.

Bernhard was a respected criminal investigator and well-known to the local society in the town where he lived and worked at the time. As his wife said, it all started one morning when he woke up telling her that he had a strange headache that he had not felt before. He could not explain this nor describe it in any detail, but it was vague, diffuse and of low intensity. They had breakfast, and he went to work and said nothing about it for some time. Then, perhaps a week or two later, he said that he felt a strange sensation, like a liquid that "sieved" over his head. She recalled him talking about the headache and asked if it was the same sensation that he had had just a few weeks before. He replied that perhaps it was. It recurred once or twice during a years' time and was then was gone. At least he did not speak about it anymore, and he did not show any other signs of being affected in any kind of way. He was 55 years old at the time and in the peak of his career as a Chief Criminal Investigator with a staff of 20 police investigators reporting to him. In the town where he worked he was known to the public due to one or two criminal cases where he had made public appearances requesting their understanding and also providing them with acceptable explanations to what was happening at the time. This was especially the case with a serial murder in which they suspected a local person as the perpetrator. He was a calm, warm and likable person and did very well in his media appearances. He appeared not only in the local press and TV but also in the national news. When the case was solved and the murderer busted, he became associated with a professional police force that always could be trusted for being focused on doing their job: he was idealized as the front figure and icon.

Bernhard's office was in the central part of town, and he was used to going into the city every morning. He usually had briefing meetings with his staff three mornings per week, depending on the load of work and complexity of the criminal cases they were working on. He was punctual and somewhat formal, and he liked to have his reports turned in on time and in good form. He usually had his door open to his staff, and everyone on his team knew what he was working on most of the time.

Therefore, what happened to Bernhard was peculiar in that one day he did not show up at the office. His staff went about doing their work, but when he had an appointment and he had not shown up, his secretary gave him a call to see if he was coming. Bernhard responded that he was late, and that he would arrive soon.

And so he did. When he arrived he apologized to the staff waiting for him. His secretary had also paved the way by bringing coffee and serving the guest waiting for him. This event went by almost unnoticed, and after a week as other stories replaced this one, no one talked about it any longer.

It might just have been a one-time event if it weren't for the fact that it actually happened again. This time Bernhard had a visitor from outside of the department, and therefore it was clearly more embarrassing to his secretary, who once again did her utmost to serve the guest and take care of any anticipatory tension. She had to call Bernhard several times since he did not respond on the first couple of attempts to reach him. Then he answered in a rather rude way by asking "Why are you calling me now?"

His secretary was a bit surprised by this response from him, but she explained that his visitor was waiting for him in his office. He then cleared his throat, as she recalled it, and said he would be there at once.

When he arrived he was not formally dressed: he had no tie and a he wore a slightly untidy shirt underneath his suit. He apologized to the guest and the meeting went by as planned with the exception of the delay. This time, his secretary was a bit annoyed and (as customary in Sweden) she took the opportunity after the meeting to ask why he was not prepared and what she could have done more to help him. He gave her a rather short and blunt answer, and she retracted to her office feeling a bit uneasy with the whole situation.

As it now had happened twice and his response to his secretary somehow leaked out, this event kicked off a discussion, a rumour, among his staff, that something was going on – something that was not yet official. He was such a respected officer and very well-liked both as a boss and an individual, so the interpretation went in the direction of logic.

The junior staff rumoured that perhaps he was attending secret meetings regarding an international assignment or perhaps collaborating with the Stockholm police force or perhaps with the secret police. Not only the junior staff, but also some seniors speculated, and with time it seemed that another rumour grew: namely, that he had meetings about the future of the department. Perhaps they were to make cuts and he could not reveal anything yet. At the same time, Bernhard's behaviour continued to change, the most evident area being affected was his punctuality for internal administrative meetings. Immediately, this led to accommodations among his direct reports and juniors who took on more responsibility for solving and covering up behind his back for issues and events that turned up in the wake of his changes. All of this occurred with the belief that bigger things were in the making.

Bernhard almost unnoticeably started to change his routines; for example, he neglected to read some emails, and occasionally he did not answer the phone while he was in his office. Sometimes he would take longer lunch breaks. It all happened so slowly, which confirmed the growing assumption among his staff who thought it was all planned and conscious changes to his routines.

It was not until perhaps a few months later that he "rudely bit someone's head off" in a conversation during an internal administrative meeting. This had never happened before, as Bernhard was recognized for being a polite boss – someone who always listened to everyone – although he could dictate, demand and drive the department in the intended professional direction without hesitation. He was a natural and charming leader, a boss that governed with gentleness. For that reason, this reaction was unprecedented, and had it not been that his staff already had made so many adaptations, they would probably have responded more outspokenly. But it all passed without any protests or reactions; instead, it increased the strength of the rumour that something was going to change in the department. The entire staff adapted and prepared for this. Bernhard did not need to apologize since they were all set up for the change to occur.

It happened again in a meeting a few weeks later and then yet another time in another meeting about one week after that. Perhaps this all could have been acceptable if it weren't for the fact that Bernhard also displayed other changes in his professional behaviour. He started to interrupt people in meetings with comments that did not always seem appropriate or professional. He commented on the dress code of some younger female staff and he began closing his door while he was in the office. He skipped some meetings without telling where he was or why he didn't show up, and the accommodations that had to be made due to these further changes became overly-stretched; it was soon impossible for his direct reports to handle them. Some of them tried to investigate what was going on and asked him straight out, only to get a nonsense reply.

The information about his changes then started to spread outside of the reporting lines, and soon Bernhard's superior was informed and called for a meeting. This should have made Bernhard start considering his manners, but not so. On the contrary, he took his new behaviour to a new level when he started interrupting others for no reason and responding with more and more illogical answers and comments. He also began taking increasingly more time off without telling where he was.

The meeting with his boss came soon afterwards. There is no record of this, but Bernhard's wife said that nothing really seemed to happen for a while: Bernhard just kept on doing what he felt was right for him. This went on for a couple of weeks until Bernhard had become completely unrecognizable. For example, he brought beer cans to his office. Finally, his boss decided to pay Bernhard a visit in his own department. His office was untidy by now, and papers lay all over the room among leftovers from lunches a few days old. It was clear that Bernhard was not well-suited for this position right now.

His Boss made a call to Bernhard's wife and asked her to take him home. He told her that Bernhard would be off duty for a while until they knew what was wrong with him. Meanwhile, he told her that, although Bernhard was highly-respected, well-liked and always welcome back, someone else would need to be assigned to do the job so that there would be no rush for Bernhard to come back. He ended the call by requesting that they meet at Bernhard's home the next day and that they contact a physician to have Bernhard go through a proper health investigation.

According to Bernhard's wife, she had also noticed how things had changed with him at home. It started with his leaving food on the table and not helping to clear dishes, and then it spread into other areas of domestic work such as taking care of the garden and the car and cleaning at home. She had tried several times to talk to him, and at first he looked surprised that she even brought it up. Later on, he began to be slightly verbally abusive and protested against her complaints. She had already noticed the change in the way that he opposed her: previously, he had always been very objective or at least had tried to be. But now, she noticed that he was clearly not trying to refer to any standards or ideals, but rather he referred to what *he* thought was best. He claimed that this was sufficient for him. Somehow he seemed more and more egoistic.

The changes with Bernhard didn't stop there: his wife also noticed that over time he had become less and less interested in how he dressed. It started out with him leaving the tie off and perhaps wearing shirts that he had used for several days already. Previously, he would have been very careful with his dressing. Over a year, the situation evolved to the state where he would go to work in clothes that he used at home to work in and spend time in while on vacation. She also noted (in keeping with this change) that he didn't care about his looks. He had always been very thorough with his hair and shaving every day, sometimes even twice, but now he just let his beard grow.

Bernhard's wife also noticed that he was becoming increasingly rude when he talked to the kids. They had two adult children, one daughter and one son, who were both starting their own family and raising children. Bernhard seemed less and less interested in talking to his children, yet before all this started, he had always been very interested in them and very attentive when they called. Now he just handed the telephone over to his wife. He could also be quite abusive and rude when speaking to them. He never even asked about the grandchildren, which was a big surprise to his wife. This was not the only change: she had also noticed that Bernhard was increasingly angry and impulsive at times, especially when he drank a little alcohol. It seemed that he couldn't tolerate any dose, but he almost immediately burst out into strange expressions, and she would get her dose of challenging (and even abusive) statements. She had thought for a long time that this had to do with his work and that he was stressed out with all the things that had happened to him there. With all the challenges of the criminal activity increasing in the town where they lived, she thought to herself that this was not a big surprise, but more what could be expected from Bernhard. After all, he was only human, and with his job's tension and stress and the potential for disaster if he wasn't successful in his job, most of these changes within him were understandable.

However, the turning point for her in defending Bernhard's behaviour came when he started to bring things home which she thought were very odd or peculiar and not fitting into their home or not at all fitting with his style. It started out with him bringing home strange food from the local store; for example, there were tins of exotic food that they never ate or candy that he never liked before. With time, Bernhard's behaviour evolved into him bringing home things such as tools that were not meant to be in a home. Bernhard explained that they could be used for gardening or working on his car in the garage. She also noticed that he brought home an increasing amount of low-alcohol beer. For a time he also seemed to buy more clothes – mostly work clothes – as if he were starting a big project at home like remodelling the attic or something.

Another strange finding was that Bernhard seemed to stay at work much longer than before. His wife knew he had a lot of responsibility at work, and she was used to him working late from time to time, especially when they had difficult cases. However, now the pattern was much more random, and he seemed to come home at unpredictable times, for example, almost at midnight or just after lunch. She could not really figure out why he had this strange pattern. When she asked him about it, he said everything was fine, and he didn't give any satisfying explanation – just a brief response.

But it was a final event that made Bernhard's wife realise that something was clearly not right: it was a phone call from the local store where they used to buy groceries. The manager of the local store called her at work to ask about her husband who, for the past couple of weeks, had made daily visits to the store just to bring home beer. Perhaps that would not be peculiar in itself, but the fact that he didn't pay anything was upsetting to them. Everybody knew who Bernhard was, a well-respected police officer in the city, and they expected the best from him and had the highest admiration for him. But still, what he did was simply a bit too much. Bernhard's wife promised to sort things out, and she immediately went to the local store and paid the debt that he had generated. She then went home to find him sitting in the kitchen just drinking beer and singing to himself. He was not very drunk, but he was clearly affected by the alcohol.

As promised, Bernhard's boss turned up for a new meeting a few days later. Bernhard's wife had taken the day off to be there to talk to him. Bernhard was somewhere in the house, but you would never know when he was about to leave or where he would go. It took his wife a few minutes to find him and to convince him to come down from the attic where he was working on something. He came down, took a few turns in the hallway, and then sat down by the kitchen table, uttering a few sentences about intrusion into his private life and that he had no time for cosy chats. He did not greet the others: he just sat down. He sighed loudly and then his boss started to speak. This is how Bernhard's wife described the meeting:

"How are you Bernhard?" asked his boss.

"I am just fine," said Bernhard.

"Well, let me tell you that I am really sorry for having to take you off duty," his boss began, but then Bernhard interrupted.

"Oh, you're sure about that?" Bernhard asked.

"Yes, I am," his boss continued. "This was inevitable, Bernhard. I would like to tell you why, but it struck me on the way coming here that I would rather like to know how you view your own way of working up till now."

"It's fine, as I said. No comments. You should just put me back to work straight away."

"So you don't think you were having any problems at work?"

"No, I am fine, I said," responded Bernhard.

"Well, for the past 6 months you have been coming late to work more and more – sometimes not turning up at all. You miss important meetings, and nobody knows where you are. You have yelled at people, and you've missed important communication from seniors such as me. You have not been able to handle your work lately. You even brought beer cans to your office. And, when I visited your office, I found it in a complete mess. Are you aware of this?"

"What do you mean? asked Bernhard.

"Don't you see anything peculiar in what I have just told you, Bernhard?"

"No, why?"

Bernhard's wife sat just quietly beside him and was saddened by Bernhard's responses. She knew he had changed a lot, but this was more than she could ever imagine about him. His boss just stared at him, waiting for some reaction, but Bernhard seemed completely unaffected by what he just had said.

"So, are we finished now?" Bernhard asked.

"Well, I would like to know what you are going to do now," his boss replied.

"What do you mean?" asked Bernhard. "I am fine."

"Well, you can't come back to work for a while, and you need to get well."

"I am not sick," said Bernhard.

"You know that you are highly respected by all your colleagues at work, but you have certainly changed so much that I think you may be ill and should see a physician."

"Hey!" shouted Bernhard without warning. "I am fine. You should not have come here since I didn't want you to," said Bernhard. "So get out of my house, now!"

"I am sorry that you feel that way since I am actually just trying to understand and help," his boss replied.

"Well, you should go home now," said Bernhard.

"Please," said his wife "He just wants you to be well."

"I am fine. You should go now," Bernhard said.

"I am sorry," said his boss looking at Bernhard's wife. "If there is anything I can do, please let me know."

Bernhard stood up abruptly and took long, swift steps out of the kitchen and began walking around in the living room. Meanwhile, his boss handed Bernhard's wife a business card with contact information and some other hand-written information on how to get into contact with his secretary and a physician that used to work closely with the police.

"You might need this," said his boss. "Feel free to call me at any time."

Then he went out in the corridor and looked for Bernhard, who by now was out in the garden. So he decided to leave the house and walk over to his car without saying goodbye to Bernhard. On his way out he could see in the reflection of his car's glass how Bernhard was pointing his finger and waiving his arm in the air as if he was threatening him. His boss did not turn around as he saw that Bernhard was somewhat ambivalent and was pacing back and forth after he went back into his garden.

A few days later, the boss called Bernhard's wife (she had given him her phone number as well). He checked on how Bernhard was doing. Bernhard's wife responded that there was no change. Bernhard wasn't speaking to her, and she guessed that perhaps he was mad at her. He was going out a lot and coming back late in the evening. She had tried several times to talk to him, but he was simply not interested in communicating with her. He just walked away when she approached him. His behaviour was also becoming stranger by the day, and his wife felt he was not normal, but she couldn't explain how. She wanted to take him to a physician, but that seemed impossible right now. His boss concluded that he would come back to her in a few days and that she could always call him if anything occurred. He would try to figure out how they could take Bernhard to a doctor.

On several occasions after the boss's visit, Bernhard looked like he was angry, and it was not long before he began yelling at his wife, especially when he came home late in the evenings. It didn't matter if she was awake or asleep: he just stormed into their bedroom, not taking notice, and then began yelling at her, sometimes even making faces and gestures that looked like he was going to smack her. His wife grew more and more cautious. She also felt an increasing sense of anxiety when she was close to him, but somehow she also denied it. She talked with the neighbours (who had done their best to avoid him for some time), and they asked her how she felt. Later that same day, Bernhard stormed at her for talking to what he called "spies and traitors". She decided to move away from home for a few days.

If it weren't for the fact that the kids already knew about Bernhard's changes, his wife probably would have chosen a hotel for a few nights' stay. But instead she drove straight to her daughter's home. They talked almost all night, crying and mourning, and the next day she called her son to tell him what was going on. The shock had passed, and now they were ready for action. They came up with a plan for how they would get Bernhard to a doctor.

The next afternoon Bernhard's wife and children all went together to try to convince him to come to his senses. They had to wait for him for several hours since he was out on one of his usual whereabouts in the city. During the wait they had time to do some cleaning up of the home as by now it had become rather messy. What they found surprised and saddened them. It turned out that Bernhard had brought home a lot of things that did not belong to them. It seemed as if he had picked up almost anything on his way home: there were empty cans, garbage, boxes of wood, magazines, garden tools, bicycle wheels and gears of all kinds. They did what they could to sort things out and clean up the mess before he arrived.

A few hours later, Bernhard made an abrupt entry, almost as if he was attacking the house in expectation of intruders.

"What is this? Who are you to come here into my house?" Bernhard shouted.

"It's us, your family, your children," said his wife.

When Bernhard saw his family he began yelling at them, asking why they were there and why they hadn't come before. He also made some strange and nonsense remarks.

"We are here because we love you," said his wife.

This did not help: Bernhard was agitated and angry. The family tried to calm him down and explained that they wanted to help. Bernhard, with a loud voice, exclaimed that he did not need any help. He said he was a "solvent and a one-man stand". This went on for about an hour, and then afterwards he left the house again. His son ran after him, trying to convince him to stay as he pulled his father's arm. This was a disaster in terms of the negotiation, but at least they all now knew something was terribly wrong with Bernhard and that they had to create a better game plan in order to get him to the hospital. This turned out to be trickier than they ever could have imagined. Telling him straight out was not an option (they had already tried that), and every attempt to trick him into following along was a failure. By this time Bernhard always went his own way.

To their great surprise and fortune, the turning point came when Bernhard caught a cold a few days later. When they were in the house one Saturday afternoon to do some more cleaning, they found him sitting on the living room sofa with a cloth around his neck, sneezing and coughing and looking all but tough. He told his wife he did not feel well and that he might be ill. Perhaps it was nothing serious, but he was not sure. The family immediately seized the opportunity to comfort and cuddle him, saying they should find out what was wrong before it became too late. (Bernhard's wife had already talked to and visited with their local physician a few times to see how he reacted to the story.) Bernhard agreed instantaneously, but he was clear that he would only go with her, not the kids. And so they went to the physician.

They didn't have to wait long at the hospital: the physician rearranged his schedule to allow for an early meeting with Bernhard. (Someone like this may decide to just leave, so you need to act while there is an opening.) As it turned out, their family physician had worked in psychiatry and immediately had a sense that this was a case that best could be helped by psychiatric intervention. Bernhard was tired and did nothing to object, nor did he try to hide the fact that he was yawning. At the same time, Bernhard complained about an illness that he felt could be serious. He asked his physician in a tone of voice that could have come from a movie:

"Is this serious doctor? Is it deadly?"

The Physician took his time to answer him about his illness, which made Bernhard look more and more worried and ill. It was as if all his powers, all his energy, suddenly went into a great big worry. He almost looked like a small child who had lost his teddy bear. Then the physician investigated Bernhard's mouth, lymph nodes, lungs and his abdomen, all during serious silence. After several minutes, the doctor once more asked how he was doing. This time Bernhard said, "I am ill, ill, very ill".

The doctor continued, "I think I need to keep you here at the hospital and let other physicians investigate you since I am not yet sure what it is. You definitely have a cold; maybe it has also affected the lungs to some extent and you have fever. But, it may be that you have something else in addition to that – something aggravating.

Bernhard agreed to stay and was taken to an internal medicine department where he soon became an irritation, a nuisance to all, and impossible to keep. He went from having a serious illness during the day to complete recovery during the night. He started stealing equipment from the nurses, trying to obstruct their work, and also stealing from his fellow patients. He was up during the night making strange noises. He easily became irritated and borderline threatening, so the nursing staff called upon a psychiatrist to investigate him. He was diagnosed with suspected psychosis and in need of immediate psychiatric care. He was then taken over to the psychiatric unit where, over a few weeks, he rapidly progressed into severe disruptive behaviour, as if the dam had broken and everything came rushing out. In just a few months Bernhard had gone from being able to at least hold a position at work (although with great difficulties) to having lost all boundaries.

Over the course of the next year, Bernhard progressed into not managing his hygiene, not following any instructions or advice, continually stealing from others, having disruptive behaviour, being abusive towards his wife and kids, and becoming very difficult to maintain, among other things. Even with specialized staff, it was difficult to manage Bernhard in a psychiatric ward, and sometimes he had to be medicated in order to keep him from harming fellow patients. Investigations of his brain were also difficult, but an MRI of the brain was done when he could be convinced that it was for medical reasons. The brain imaging showed a severe orbitofrontal degeneration of the brain, meaning that the parts of the brain that are located just above the nose were severely affected. This type of brain degeneration may be due to Alzheimer's disease, but more commonly it is seen in frontotemporal lobe dementia, which is a group of disorders with a common trait of brain degeneration. It may sometimes be seen in ALS, bipolar disorder and schizophrenia as well.

Bernhard was placed in a special care unit as the only patient with an all-male staff around to guard him since he was abusive to women. For over two years it was almost impossible for his family to visit him due to him becoming aggressive. At the same time, his speech changed into expressing fewer and fewer words, repeating phrases and making illogical statements. He still found his way around, however, and he kept trying to steal and hoard things. His strength and trained physical skills made his care challenging for the staff. He also began putting various things in his mouth, as if regressing to a child's level of eating everything from dust to dirt. Eventually, Bernhard died of pneumonia.

While he was kept in the special care unit, his wife found a lot of things that Bernhard had collected and brought home and she felt uneasy with having all this in the house. She decided to call Bernhard's boss and asked for a special investigation to be made on the goods. A few days later, a police officer was assigned to go through the things before sending it to a local storage facility. It took him a few days to sort things out. Among the things he identified were garden tools, pieces of wood and plastic, papers, bags, cans and tools, and some electronics. One of the more interesting things was a mobile phone with a pay card. At first the idea was to get rid of all things Bernhard had collected, but then the officer had a gut feeling that he should send the mobile phone to a forensic lab for further investigation. It took more than a month to get any response from the lab, but afterwards he received a phone call and then a letter stating that the lab had found some interesting calls made to numbers that had been linked to a gold and diamond store heist about a year ago. Previously, the police only had loose ends, but with this phone, they could connect the dots and make an explanation out of all the data. Besides the data and the calls made, they had also found finger prints that not only belonged to Bernhard, but also to one of the neighbours a couple of houses further down the road from Bernhard. Having this as a piece of evidence, a chain of findings that initially seemed random could be linked together, and a search warrant could be made for the neighbour's house where the police collected further evidence linking the neighbour to the robbery. When Bernhard died, the story was revealed, and at the time of the funeral, Bernhard was once again a hero. If it weren't for him the case would not have been solved. It seemed that Bernhard, in spite of his whereabouts during his illness (until the bitter and dramatic end), would stay useful to the corps. As they say, "Once an officer, always an officer."

7 THE REFLEX MAN

On one particular day, I recall that I had a completely full agenda with patients from early morning to late in the afternoon, which included several new patients to be interviewed and investigated. As so many times before, I ate my lunch in my office and had basically no time for anything else but patients, so dictations that needed to be made were piling up.

Reaching the end of the day, I brought a cup of coffee with me while walking towards the waiting room. The coffee was hot and strong from synthetic oils and caffeine, and I finished it just before I opened the door. I noticed the waiting room was unusually empty except for one man who sat near the door looking at me with clear blue, wide-open, almost-staring eyes. I asked his name, and he quickly confirmed that he was to visit me. I noticed while talking to him that he was exceptionally well-dressed and also had well-groomed hair; it almost looked as if it were dyed.

As was the custom, we went together to my office, and he walked beside me through the corridor. That day we had to make our way through a group of medical students who, during their break from a lecture, chatted with each other in a quite noisy way, almost as if they felt nervous. Some lectures in psychiatry usually provoked reactions and brought about nervous behaviours from the young adults who still had a long way to go before they were ready to face the realities of a medical practice of their own.

As we got into my office, my patient (who was called Joshua) immediately started into his story as if he were bursting to tell it, not being able to hold it back any longer. Joshua told me he was 37 years old and had lived with another man for a couple of years. He had tried different relationships: in the beginning he lived for a short while with a woman, but it was obvious to him from early on that he felt deep inside himself that he longed for the love of a man. Joshua was an educated teacher at the University, having a temporary position there while working on a thesis in literature.

In spite of being born in a country where the acceptance of homosexuality was low, Joshua was by now a fully-assimilated Swede and spoke fluently without any noticeable accent. It had been almost 30 years since he, his mother and brother had arrived here, and although the start was rough and almost tore them apart, they were all now established and in balance with their new environment. Joshua was confident when he said that he was a calm and serious person, but he added that he also liked to have fun "shaking in the sun", bursting out in a high-pitched seizure-like, and almost jerky type of laughter. It was quite unique to him and was not a type of glee that would immediately invite someone to join, but rather stop and observe what was going on. This jerkiness came back without any warning a couple of times in our conversation and was always preceded by a short witty statement. It seemed to me that he was making jokes out of a word, or part of a word, or even a sound from the expression of a word. On occasion, he even made jokes about noises, not really trying to imitate them, but rather capture or describe a part of the noise in a witty way.

Joshua was remarkable in many ways. I especially noticed this the first I saw him, but he presented new characteristics every time we met. What happened during this first meeting was in reality quite spectacular, but due to his capabilities, it all went by almost unnoticed. As he spoke about himself, he suddenly started to describe something while waving his hand in the air. As he did this, he accidently touched a small vase that was standing on the table in front of us, and it started to fall to the ground. However: Joshua managed to continue his movement, and with very fast reflexes, he caught the vase in his hand, just before it was to reach the ground. He then just continued to talk like it was the most natural thing in the world. I was quite astonished with this and at the same time unruffled since it had happened so fast while he was completely focused on the story he told. It was almost as if it didn't happen at all, and Joshua just continued. Maybe his tempo increased somewhat, but it was already quite fast from the start; this must have been normal for him. This was his habitual state of mind.

To Joshua, the wittiness was something he was proud of and which he thought also helped him to build social relations. However, he was also painfully aware that it seemed to bring him, at least on some occasions, into more difficult situations as exemplified when he was the only one laughing and everyone else was just watching. It had never really bothered him much since he really liked his own laughter, but since he had gotten negative feedback from his headmaster, his boss, it was very clear now also to him that something was very wrong. He had been told that his jokes were sometimes inappropriate, and when teaching at the University, it caused confusion among his students, as they were outspoken about their education and teachers, especially the young ones. With time, it led to a build-up of attitudes and notions about him as a person, about his style and eventually also about his intelligence. The academic world is in many ways formal, and attitudes are, more often than not, stale and rigid with a tendency towards low tolerance for extremes. The eccentric typically do not succeed academically; otherwise it all would lead to the opposite reaction, namely acceptance and admiration. And so, becoming a successful teacher in the academic world means you would either need to adapt to or change the system to survive. Adapting is far easier.

Joshua was at the height of his academic career, and the future could either look very bright or, if things went wrong, just terrible. It was clear that he was concerned, but the way in which he talked about it might cause a person to think that he was careless and easy-going about it. He wore a casual, almost goofy smile and said that he probably just had a "tilted mind" and that he might even be abnormal. He then added that it would be good to know just in case he was suffering from ADHD or something like that, since then he would have an excuse for his boss.

He turned his gaze away and stopped talking for just a few seconds. I almost had time to start thinking about where he was heading. He looked a bit sad, and then he said his behaviour had been going on for so many years, as long as he could remember, and yet it just started giving him trouble. Still looking away he continued with, "It would be easier if I could just understand why they reacted to me." It was evident that he was affected by all the negative feedback.

I asked about his teaching, which brought an immediate response. He moved around a little before he started, as if he was preparing for a physical activity.

"You know, I have a rather strict scheme," he said. Then he talked for several minutes about how he structured his lectures. It was evident that this was very important to him: he talked and talked about it. I am not even sure that he was aware of whether I was listening or not; he seemed completely absorbed in the matter.

In fact, overall, structure seemed to be essential in his life, and any deviation from this pattern caused stress and anxiety within him. Repetition helped him keep himself together, it seemed. Lectures had to follow this strict pattern, and questions would be allowed only at the end of the session. He thought he was regarded as a good teacher, and that made it even harder for him to grasp why he had received this critique.

We reached the end of the session and it was almost difficult for him to round-up his description of his structures, and in spite of my cautious mentioning of the time of the day, he seemed rather pleased with the meeting. Before he left I gave him a task to consider before the next time. I suggested he would observe and make note of situations in which others did not react as he expected. He willingly accepted this being the receptive learner he was.

In-between the first and second sessions, my thoughts went several times to this Joshua and his dilemma. I began to construct a theory of his jocularity. In the context of his almost-obsessive need for structure, there was a fear that if he could not control his environment he would have an outburst. Noticeable structure and deliberate repetition were essential. Energy was present and was a valuable source of power and success. Low energy, lack of structure, and changes were hazards. At the same time, while staying out of danger, the energy led to the accumulation of tension inside, which after a while needed a release like steam searching for a pipe in order to escape; it was a release of inner pressure. The jokes were like a cork to be ejected, like a long-stored bottle of champagne in urgent need of drinking. Suddenly it all bubbled up, relieving him of tensions that had built up while holding on to all the routines, all the structures and the repetition.

The next session started in the same fashion as the first had with Joshua bursting out into describing his situation, and this time it included the mentioning of his homework. While he eagerly continued to talk about the importance of his structures, not giving any substantial examples of observations that he had made, I took the risk of causing confusion and interrupted him in his long speech. I asked him if he felt any tension inside while working. He just stopped in the middle of a sentence and held his breath for what seemed like a minute, and then he breathed out loudly, letting all his muscles unwind.

"Yes," was the first word that came out. "Oh yes," then followed. "I always feel a lot of pressure," he continued. "It has been following me ever since I was born," he said. He was again quiet for a minute or two, and I just let him rest for a moment. The question and the revealed insight had put him out of balance. He asked for a glass of water. Contemplation had taken over. Water, air, light, sounds of silence – the basic elements provided comfort. Joshua was relaxed in a way I had never seen him before.

The session ended. I followed Joshua out of the building, which by now was empty, except for the cleaning staff which seemed to have a preference for staying in the shadows, silently, rhythmically wiping off what the day had brought. I asked if he needed help with transportation, but Joshua's only response was, "Thanks," while he shook his head.

We set up his next appointment, but I wasn't sure if he would return. Perhaps this had been too much for him. Perhaps he was scared to lose it all, thinking that I would continue to manipulate him out of his powers. I was concerned and considered calling him. The session played over and over in my mind that evening, but time went by, other patients caught my attention and the nagging impression of that session slowly faded away.

The day arrived when he was to return, and I had worked on lowering my expectations. Joshua sat there looking at me with the same eyes, in the same spot, at the same time in the usual empty waiting room. The room to the lecture hall was closed as we passed it this time; there were no restless medical students in the area. We didn't speak on the way over to my room. Things would turn out to be the same, however, since as soon as I closed the door to my room he immediately started to speak. He said he had thought a lot about what he had felt that previous session. It was a bullet through his heart, he said. It had opened up his awareness of how governed he was by his inner tension and how this was so closely intertwined with his need for control. He had been unusually quiet, his boyfriend had told him, for several days. He also told me had been sleeping poorly, perhaps just a few hours a night, waking up early and feeling stressed and worn out. The first few days after our talk he had a headache. It was a chronic type of tension like a band of metal that would not let go being strapped around his forehead. At the same time he was fully aware that what we had talked about was completely relevant to him. The tension in his life had been present for as long as he could remember. There were long episodes when he did not recognize it. He lived (or he felt like he lived) a normal life, but then he eventually reached a stage where it caught up with him, perhaps after a few weeks, and he suddenly felt completely exhausted. "I could not manage to do anything for a couple of days," he said.

As he grew older, he had realized that his exhaustion had to do with that inner tension that he felt. Even though he had thought about how to get rid of the tension and even tried various strategies like meditation, muscle relaxation and even exercise, nothing seem to relieve him of this pressure. At the same time, he was convinced that this tension was directly correlated to his performance and that if he would somehow find a way to get rid of it, it would have a negative impact on his capacity and perhaps counteract his performance and his career.

I asked him if he had spoken to anyone before about his tension, and his immediate response was, "No." He said he realized later on that his partner had made jokes about him, especially when he got into his periods of exhaustion, but that his own awareness of his issue had only come about the last few days after we had spoken. He trusted his roommate, his lifelong friend and partner, with so many things, but this was more of a secret – something deep within him, and he almost seemed to have a mystic hunch involving this inner tension that if he would ever speak to someone about it, he would lose all the magical strength that he felt he had. However, now it was inevitable that he give up this idea, and he was ready, for the first time in his life, to open up.

I asked him how he felt about it, and he said it was a mixed bag of pain and relief. He was plagued by the conviction that it would rob him of some of his magic, but at the same time he felt strongly that he had to do something about it. We talked for nearly an hour about this tension, trying to map when, where, how, and in which situations he had the strongest inner tension, and when, how and what he did to feel the strongest relief from it. He used a paper and pencil as he worked his way through drawings, maps, and charts to uncover patterns. This was something that he liked and mastered: it made his magic concrete and visual.

After this first session about his tension, Joshua told me he was relieved that we had talked about it. The next time he came back for a session, it was clear that he was much more positive, and he immediately wanted to continue the charting. We continued to map his inner and outer landscape trying to reach his automatic thoughts, feelings, and behaviours, working according to a basic cognitive behavioural therapeutic model.

That was a time in my career when I underwent supervision training to master the first step of cognitive therapy, and I was blessed with an excellent tutor, one of the founding mothers of CBT in Sweden, who guided me with such an ease and knowledge, making each training session a revelation. For Joshua, this meant that he began to undertake an almost scientific approach to his tension, and even though it was not the plan from the start, it became a catalyst that made it possible for Joshua to come back with another tactic, another method and optimism to re-focus on his jocularity and his reflex responses that had been the reason for coming to me from the start.

We focused perhaps three sessions on his inner tension, but then Joshua was ready to go back to the initial topic: his jocularity. Using his regained motivation and his optimism, we started to charter and map the where's, the how's, the when's and in which situations it all appeared, focusing on his attention, making him a scientist investigating his own thoughts and awareness as well as other people's reactions and responses. I stressed that he shouldn't try to change, but just continue to be the one he had always been and observe others as he began his exploration. I advised him to let his boss know of the progress he made and that he was in the exploration mode, so he should not expect any swift changes. He thought it was an excellent idea.

Coming back to the next session, I could tell that he was even more confident than before, and now he was also a believer in progress related to his personal issues. Joshua was a clever explorer and an excellent scientist, and perhaps was it due to a combination of both his verbal intelligence and his already-acquired capability of sticking to routines that he made swift progress.

Joshua's jocularity depicts his dilemma, as it was both the way in which he would make a joke, and then his issue with understanding, or rather lack of understanding, of how others perceived his joke in that particular context. The joke in itself would in some instances be perceived as funny or even hilarious, and the example above especially illustrates how Joshua usually created his jokes, namely by a form of word-alliteration and paronomasia[20]. Thus, by using or playing with similarly sounding words, he switched the context of a sentence to something he perceived as funny. This paronomasia was characteristic of his jokes and also was evident in his professional writing where he unintentionally overused this rhetorical method. Someone reading his papers or articles would find this emerging as his signature, of sorts. When this was brought up in a subsequent session, he was first surprised and claimed he was unaware of this tendency. He then denied it as being something he did consciously. He also insisted that it was *not* that pregnant in his writing, and he gave examples of other rhetorical methods that he used.

Joshua also displayed some other signs indicative of his issues. He had problems in perceiving differences between himself and others. You could say he thought that he was like everyone else (i.e., he believed that his thoughts represented what is normal or the standard.) This means he did not start by thinking what others may perceive of a situation or that they would indeed see something differently than he did. You may call this a preference

---

[20] http://en.wiktionary.org/wiki/paronomasia

of perspective or, if you would like, a self-centred perspective. In our further discussions I found out that he indeed could be caring and considerate, but when he spoke or wrote he had a strong preference for promoting his own point of view. An alternative way of viewing Joshua's difficulties would be that he had a weakness in empathetic thinking, at least when he spoke or wrote, or it could be seen as a sign of weakness in the ability to generate an immediate hypothesis about other people's thinking (what sometimes is called "theory of mind").

At the next session, Joshua came back and told me that he focused almost completely on other people's reactions, and then slowly began to notice differences between the situations where he was amongst his loved ones, his friends, and when being at work. This was a great sign of insight being developed in Joshua. He started in a very elaborate way to explore the differences between his home and work life. In the same manner that he explored his own awareness, he told me that it was very difficult for him to switch his attention from, as he said, "describing with words and pictures to studying the images of others" as he was speaking. What he meant was the images of other people's faces as they listened to him, expressing various emotions and reactions to what he said. This may be hard in general, but for Joshua this turned out to be the trickiest part and the one that held him back from understanding the interplay between people. We worked on his change in attention – his focus on his own awareness. I gave him exercises, and he practiced them when we met. Eventually he made progress.

One day he came back telling about what he had noticed in others. It was a great moment for Joshua as he also told me he was able to understand these experiences that he felt others had to things that he said, noticing the difference between factual discussions and when he made a joke. He went as far in his exploration as to ask two of his most trusted colleagues what they thought about his sense of humour and was fortunate that they both were glad to share their reflections. Probably, they had noticed it for a long time and were potentially aware that it was an issue. What he learnt was the impression they had was that his jokes often came very abruptly, not always fitting the situation, and that it then often became awkward. However, they were also very clear in saying that the same type of jokes would fit in well in another setting, perhaps at a pub or a cocktail party. This was vital feedback to Joshua, and after this feedback he started to explore variations in his interactions, not only with the students, but also with his colleagues, gaining valuable insights into how people reacted to him. I encouraged him to be patient and stick to his plan since it would probably take a while before he noticed a clear change in other people's reactions and also before he would feel more confident in his newly-acquired skills.

Being the good student, Joshua undertook a few weeks of practice where, in fact, he didn't come back on the regular basis, but just updated me via brief telephone calls. Instead, we planned a new pair of sessions a month later where we would use his results to begin to focus on exploring alternative approaches and behaviours for him.

It turned out that this pause in our sessions and Joshua's focusing for a longer time on the exploration was a successful approach for him. He became more and more confident and also found ways to manage his tension. He also gained confidence in being able to master the approach to learning about himself and ways to modify how he interacted with other people.

When he came back to me for what turned out to be the last session, he wanted to know what it all could have been (talking in terms of a diagnosis). I told him that what he was experiencing, the jocularity, his almost obsessiveness with routines, his inner tension and especially the way in which he made jokes (all of which were still present in him, but were being managed by amore evident self-control and self-distance), could be described as anxiety, as in obsessive-compulsiveness, but perhaps better described as part of the spectrum of Tourette's syndrome. In view of his capacity and ability to deal with his issues, and also in view of the original signs and symptoms (the swift reflexes, his obsessiveness, his jocularity, his language puns and his somewhat disinhibited jokes) it pointed to something that would lie within the spectrum of a Tourette syndrome. I told Joshua that would characterize it as a light version of Tourette: Tourette's Light.

To my surprise, Joshua was almost happy to hear about this. The combination of him being intelligent, verbal, quick in responses, and now with his newly acquired self-exploring abilities, he felt that it was more or less a kind of blessing to have this diagnosis. Even though I told him he would find that if he would meet other people with Tourette syndrome he may differ quite a lot from them, he said that didn't bother him: the diagnosis itself was a relief to him. Now, he could better understand why he behaved the way he did, why his mind worked the way it did, and why people reacted as they did. Now he saw his obsessiveness in a new light.

All in all, Joshua would turn out to be both a successful student of his own abilities and of others' reactions as well as a successful therapy patient. He was someone that I myself felt I had followed side-by-side through his pains, revelations and finally reliefs into becoming a kind of master of his own abilities, of his own thinking and behaviour. Joshua would not come back to me, but he wrote me a letter after a few months talking about how happy he was that he attended the therapy sessions and gained these insights. He had also had several talks with his headmaster who had also noticed what progress he had made, and he was now approaching a period where he was to focus on preparing his thesis. Before, he had felt a lot of anxiety around it, but now he was much more confident that he would be able not only to manage to collect all his results and notes into writing a book, but also present it as a work of science. His relations with his colleagues had improved, and now he felt he was a popular teacher among the students. He wrote that he usually started his sessions by telling them that they would need to be prepared for his special sense of humour, and that they should not be worried or afraid because it was due to his suffering from a syndrome called Tourette's Light. They would not be contaminated, and they could just continue to interact with him as they wished. This was usually an ice breaker, and when the students were introduced to him in this new way, they all seemed to find better ways to interact and communicate, and the feedback from his teaching sessions improved.

Joshua was very happy with the explanation I provided. It made sense to him, which was of main importance. His dilemma, the Tourette's Light, may be viewed as part of the normal spectrum of human psychological phenotypes and is not as uncommon as one may think. However, sometimes it arises as sign of a brain lesion, often with a focus in the right frontal lobe (among left brain hemisphere dominant persons i.e. usually being right handed). Individuals who have suffered a stroke, have had a brain infection, or have had the surgical removal of a brain tumour in the right frontal lobe often develop a tendency to have a flat temperament and may appear indifferent or euphoric. They often show signs of inappropriate jocularity, or "Witzelsucht", as the German term is for this phenomena. This sign of right frontal brain dysfunction underlies different types of what may be called an impulsive or disinhibited tendency for bad jokes, corny puns, and odd behaviour. It has been labelled the "joking disease," although it is not a disease per se, but rather a symptom or sign of a dysfunction of the right side or part of the frontal brain.

Jocularity is just one of the signs that may arise from a right frontal brain lesion: loss of context, for example in social situations such as conversations, is another such sign. The loss of context is expressed as talking or behaving in a manner that is perceived as different or strange in relation to the particular situation or topic of conversation. A person with a right frontal lesion usually misses the context or is unable to read the context and will be regarded as strange. Starting to make jokes in a serious setting, for example at a funeral or in a court hearing, or making faces at a distant acquaintance with whom they are speaking, or starting to sing at a lecture when sitting in the audience, are just a few examples of this lack of context. It may be viewed as, again, a sign of a lack of inhibition, but it can also be explained by having lost the ability to read the context. Another typical sign of right frontal lobe lesion is restlessness, which may be part of this spectrum of frontal signs.

One may speculate as to how this paronomasia arises. It may be due to one of the following underlying causes: a) a lack of inhibitory control; a function that is sub-served by the right frontal lobe, in combination with, b) a loss of context of what is appropriate within a particular situation, which may be explained by a loss of inner guidance to enable one to stay within the frames of a conversation, and, c) a lack of flexibility which makes someone hold to one strategy for generating words, which together with an, d) increased release or flow of words (increased word generation), and sometimes a word creativity, would give rise to the symptoms that Joshua demonstrated.

All of the functions described above have been observed in patients who have lesions or evidence of a dysfunction in the right frontal lobe when the dominant hemisphere is the left (that is they are usually right-handed). There are several such disorders, and one of them is Tourette syndrome. Such a syndrome may not be full-fledged, but a person may suffer from part of it, which is why Tourette and other similar disorders are called spectrum disorders. What they share is that they all have their neuronal basis for their symptoms and signs in the right frontal lobe.

For Joshua, it was the diagnosis and the explanation of how his brain worked that did the trick. He himself regained his self-confidence and became an explorer of his and other persons' behaviours and reactions, something that made all the difference and led to a successful outcome for Joshua. Today, he is a recognized scientist in his field of research and still a teacher, and as I have heard, a very popular one.

Dr. Magnus Sjögren

8 SHADOWS FOLLOWED HER

What should you believe in? Should you believe only in what you experience yourself, or is it relevant to believe in what others tell you? Since you cannot really experience everything yourself, at some point you will have make a decision whether you should believe in what other people tell you or not. You probably develop a reference base to compare with and do an internal check of whether something you hear may be true or not. But there are situations and information that you lack a reference base for, and so you will need to decide if it is true or not based on something else: perhaps a gut feeling, the trustworthiness of the other person, a logical estimation of whether or not it could be true, or based on whether you want to believe it. Perhaps it is a mix of all these factors that determines whether you say, "Yes, I believe in it," or, "No, this can't be true."

Today, being sceptical is a good starting position since there is so much new information and facts that we are exposed to, and that amount seems to increase every day. We don't have a reference base for much of it, and so many things that we hear and see pass us by unnoticed: we just can't fit it into our reference base. We may say, "So what?" or simply nothing at all. Our filters are up. We don't take it in; it's not relevant, so we don't see it.

But imagine if you were the only one that had an experience – something that is so real that it just can't be ignored – something that also repeats itself making it impossible to disregard. What if your filters are down and you cannot abandon the thought of it being there, it being so real that it simply cannot be denied? And so it is your own experience, and it's all true; what others are saying won't change your belief that it is true, but it may hurt your feelings if they don't agree with you. If it becomes important to you to have the acknowledgement of others, and if this is difficult to get, such an experience may tend to make you lonely. With the repeated exposure and the refusal of others to see it, you are constantly negatively affected. No one believes you. You may think and feel that you are fighting for your life while others think you are chasing windmills. If it becomes chronic and starts affecting your life, your work, and your social behaviour, it may be as severe as to qualify as a disorder. You have become ill based on your beliefs. Delusions are within the domain of beliefs that both make you lonely and increase your risk of becoming ill. This story is about one of those many lonely persons.

Caroline grew up in Lidkoping, one of the major cities of Sweden. She attended school, and although she didn't find a lot of pleasure in the school subjects, she performed well and especially enjoyed language, history and art. She was clearly into the aesthetic subjects. She had a few friends and became interested in horse riding early in life. When she was between eleven and seventeen years old, she spent most weekends in the stable taking care of the horses. Caroline became especially good at horse racing; she was competitive and enjoyed it a lot. During her teenage years, especially in the early ones, she attended a lot of horse races and dreamed about competing on a professional level. She was never to fulfil those dreams for various reasons, a major one being the demand from her parents to acquire an education as well as the fact that horse riding was not a sport for an adult.

"This is not something you can do for a living. We know this from experience, so you'd better learn from us," was their repeated comment when she talked about her dream. They had, of course, never given their own dreams a chance, but Caroline never challenged her parents, at least not on this topic. This all led to the first of her repeated break downs – crises that recurred once or twice a year for most of her life.

During her high school years Caroline met her first boyfriend – her first lasting relationship outside the family. He was a stable boy working for pay and not really very interested in horses. Girls, on the other hand, were more his flavour, and what Caroline didn't know was that he flirted behind her back throughout their relationship. For Caroline, this love affair was a big deal, and she was very attracted to him for a long time until they broke up, which was yet another disappointment for her. The day she found out that he flirted with other girls she fell apart completely. He had broken her heart and betrayed the trust that she felt in him. She had never been as hurt before and was completely devastated. He apologized, but it was too late. They had broken their bond, and the magic was gone.

During this second major crisis in her life, Caroline began to lose her close tie to horse riding. It was as if all her hopes and beliefs deep in the core of her soul were hurt. For a long time she didn't want to do much of anything. She spent most of her spare time indoors in her bedroom talking to herself and listening to the music of Joni Mitchell. It took several months before she re-gained some signs of energy. After this she was changed. She toughened up, at least on the surface, and started to mix with questionable characters, learning how to drink and smoke. She had several brief relationships – none lasting more than a few weeks. She challenged her parents with her talk, her misconduct and her poor self-discipline. At age twenty, she moved away from her parents and lived with friends for a couple of months until she found a youth group that rented a house outside of Lidkoping where she was offered a room for low rent.

Soon thereafter Caroline got a part-time job in the city. Her new friends helped her get it. She soon was seen helping out in a store playing a rather low-keyed role, but at least she was earning a salary so that she could continue her independence. For a time, all she did was work, smoke, read and meet with a few friends. Her behaviour had slowly changed from the stormy, provocative, late-teenage days, and she had become more interested in her inner life – sharing her thoughts with just a few close companions. Her longing for knowledge came quite naturally, and she soon started to apply for courses at the University. Combining part-time jobs and studies for a few years enabled her to graduate with a bachelor's degree in social science. With that, her opportunities grew for a chance to take on positions with a higher salary. Not long afterwards she was offered a job at a high school as second counsellor. At the time, she was about 25 years old and had had a few brief relationships, but it was here, at work, that she met the Thomas, the man who would become her husband.

The two seemed to be made for each other, sharing the same interests in art and philosophy, talking for hours about concepts of the mind, perspectives on sculpture and interpretations of drawings. They had a great time together, and their love was intense. Almost anything seemed possible, and their life was full of pleasures. It wasn't long before they began living together. He was a math teacher, and she was a counsellor. The future seemed full of opportunities, and Caroline started slowly, although not fully consciously, to believe that some dreams may come true after all.

Within three years they had their first child, and after five years they had a second. They were inseparable, and their dreams grew, painting the picture of a future with more kids, a big house in the countryside, their own farm, traveling, enjoying and living life as it should be. The only thing that differed between them was that she was quite a heavy smoker and he was not. Thomas had never in his life felt attracted to smoking, but for a while his huge passion for her included the smoke that tainted her skin. The smoking was, however, to become an issue with time.

When the first years of intense love were replaced by the more sober partnership / love and friendship combo, Caroline had to find a strategy for blending her smoking in with the family's desires. She went outside to have a smoke, she washed her clothes – more often than all of theirs – over and over to make sure she shed any faint hint of smoke that could evoke a discussion. She never bought cigarettes in front of her family, and she used more and more filtered cigarettes. Her smoking became an issue when she went into her mood swings with bad self-esteem and low energy. It was then that she got sloppy and occasionally exposed her family to the side-effects of her smoking. For several years this was fine, and she and the family coped with it. However, in time her habit would grow from a bagatelle to a matter of sheer conflict, and her habitual, well-grounded sense of loneliness that she had known from childhood would re-emerge. It began to plague her and influence her image within the family as well as her image of herself in relation to them. She was different. She was lonely.

In hindsight, the first ten years of Caroline's relationship and family life were great. There was much joy, love and shared interests. They had friends, were active at the school and travelled during holidays. This initially-minor issue of her smoking habit grew ever-so slowly, and when the kids had both started primary school, it was just a black feather – still almost weightless, but evidently noticeable. Five years later it had grown into a rotten potato, and after yet another five years with both kids in their teenage years, they had a black swan in their family.

At the same time, Caroline's personality somehow changed. Bit by bit, her view of herself as an outsider grew, and her thoughts would more and more often walk the path of a stranger. She unconsciously pictured herself in situations where she was alone with no allies, where no one understood her and she had to fight harder and harder to be heard. She had occasional nightmares that grew into horrors before going to bed. Her sleep consequently worsened, and she experienced repeated interruptions. This made her tired, and she began struggling more and more often with the routines of everyday life.

The first sign that something was radically changing in Caroline was when she started to believe that Thomas had a relationship with another woman. Their kids were in their late teens, and they had almost lived together for fifteen years. It happened that he came home from work and she got a peculiar but distinct sense that he smelled differently. Caroline intuitively and immediately associated this with his having spent time with another woman. She asked him where he had been and what he had done. Thomas was surprised by her questions. Throughout their entire relationship he had never experienced her being like this; she had never challenged his credibility in this manner. The discussion quickly ended up in an argument and her notion was firm as a rock and could not be changed. She stuck with this belief, and they quarrelled every evening for about a week until the issue started to fade away. But the impression Caroline had was permanent, and time would not heal this wound in her. On the surface a time of resentment and resolution commenced, but in her mind, Thomas, her true love and beloved husband, had been with another woman in spite of him denying it all the way to the bitter end.

A few months passed, and summer entered into their life. It was a particularly sunny and warm June, and all seemed fine as they planned their holiday with joy and a sense of belonging. It seemed as if everything was as it always had been, and they were back to their roots. They went to a holiday camp in the south of France, close to Nice, where they had booked an apartment, complete with a shared pool for two weeks. There were several other families in the pool area – including young adults – who gathered around the pool every day and evening for swimming, playing with their kids and also for showing off, flirting, competing and just mingling. This was an obvious place for the seeds of family conflict. A mixture of people from different countries, different ages, different preferences and styles came together in a tiny spot. From morning till evening, with small breaks for beverages and food, they found their positions around the pool and chatted, contemplated, played, slept, and doomed each other.

For Caroline this was a clear source of concern, and she began unconsciously generating hypotheses and unshared thoughts about Thomas and others; it did not take long before she started to feel jealous of him for his easy way which opened the door for others to start chatting with him. Any time a woman said something to Thomas (which on the whole was not that often), Caroline's mind went ballistic. Just a few nights into their visit she started to accuse him of flirting, and after yet another few days she said he deliberately was trying to invite other women to have an affair with him behind her back. They quarrelled almost every night on this holiday. The kids were almost grown-up by now and had gotten used to the occasional arguments, but this time it was somewhat different. They thought their mother was strange – changed in a sad way. They could not agree with her, and when she asked them to take her side they kindly explained that they could not see it the way she did. They were embarrassed, and Thomas was sad and angry. Caroline was lonely and convinced that she was right.

This holiday cut a severe wound in their relationship, and it wasn't long after they came back that Thomas felt that they had become too distant from each other and that the once so-warm and beautiful love they had felt for each other was now almost dead. He still had feelings for Caroline but could not stand all the accusations. He tried to talk to her over and over again but she seemed so distant – as if she had vanished into deep darkness. One year later they had separated, and after two years they were divorced. Everything he did added to her beliefs of his misdoings, building up a stack of proofs that he was unfaithful and cold-hearted.

Caroline's belief about Thomas was unbreakable and laid the foundation for further misbeliefs. She grew into becoming more prone to misunderstandings and had developed a cognitive structure where everyday communication could potentially be misinterpreted, and lead to conflict. At work, she more and more often got the impression that others were trying to take her job away, that they talked behind her back and that her boss was not happy with her performance. She nurtured this thought, and it grew within her to the point that she actually, went to ask him if he was unhappy with her performance in-between one of the regular development talks. Her boss was completely taken by surprise. As he had never had this thought, he just gave her the short answer that, no, he had never thought about it. But this sudden and emotional reaction of hers made him more observant of her performance in spite of him not having any rationale of ever considering it as an issue.

Caroline, however, was not happy with his response. Since the boss was eager to have a good relationship with his team, he called her to a meeting and brought it up – kindly at first – but after her defensive reaction, he became a bit more challenging and asked her what in the world could ever underlie such a notion of hers. Caroline was already defensive, and her inner tension increased during the meeting. The boss' plan was to clear the air and calm her, but the result was just the opposite. She told him she felt convinced that he had been watching her work and that she had the impression he was rating her. She put this into a framework of on-going rationalizations at work, and she thought perhaps he planned to cut back and get rid of her. He told her that he had no reason at all to be unhappy with her, but he was surprised that she was so "suspicious". The word echoed in her mind and a flood of emotions rose within her leading to the inevitable: she began to cry. Her boss reacted instinctively and reached out to touch her, which led to her reflexive withdrawal. She regressed into her teenage position: lonely, abandoned, and accused.

When Caroline came home, the word "suspicious" echoed in her mind. She felt that her boss was angry with her and that he, as a boss, was not truly honest. This thought grew in her mind to a point where she started to feel that she was being observed and criticized, making her more and more unhappy. She decided to take a few days off for sick-leave which, in reality, meant she lay on her bed completely paralyzed with sorrow and inner pain.

When she went back to work, it seemed as though everything had changed, and she would never regain her once-excellent drive and enthusiasm. It hindered her performance, and she began having difficulties concentrating on her meetings. She fell more and more behind in her reports. Nearly every task became difficult, and eventually her boss decided to take her off duty, which worsened the situation even more. Various attempts were made to reach out to her, but she fell into what was regarded as a depression which eventually would be the first step towards a premature retirement.

I worked at the hospital in Gothenburg at the state-of-the-art psychiatric unit which had a great reputation for combining biological psychiatry with a cognitive approach in a modern environment. It offered rooms that were furnished and coloured in a delightful way making it as similar to a hotel or even to a part-time home as possible. Patients who knew the differences between the psychiatric units in the region preferred to be treated at the Gothenburg unit. It was said that it had the charm and atmosphere of a small town unit with the competence and ambition of a big town unit. For Caroline, it probably did not matter where she stayed, and the fact that she had been at the Gothenburg unit was more of a defeat to her.

She had followed the advice of her best friend and her daughter and visited the emergency unit at the hospital where a doctor suggested that she stay a few nights to map her concerns, to see how she could be helped and to possibly try medication. She unwillingly agreed to stay there for one night only since she was so very tired, not having slept for several nights. By the next morning she decided to leave. There was no review of her situation, no discussion about her needs, nor any other support besides an offer to see a psychiatrist in a non-institutional care setting in the next week. For some reason, Caroline accepted this, and she decided to see the psychiatrist, which to her was against her own principles since she did not think she was ill at all and had little hope that a physician could ever help her.

It was a typically grey and cold autumn day, and I had a temporary assignment at the non-institutional care part of psychiatry in the Gothenburg region where Caroline sat in the waiting room to see me. She was thin and looked a bit greyish as if she just had recovered from a period of illness. She was coughing lightly, which would turn out to be due to pulmonary emphysema, something she had acquired due to the many years of heavy smoking. At first she addressed my welcoming approach in a proper way, but that, along with some brief information about her, would turn out to be all that she was prepared to share with me at this first meeting.

Our first meeting could actually be described as a sort of defence game where any question I asked was met with a formally correct attitude, but emotionally and personally she resisted passing any information to me concerning her mental health. I decided at this first meeting to do all I could to give her a sense of winning this game, and at least on this first aim I succeeded, since she actually came back to me maybe three times all together. In addition, I was to meet her daughter who had asked her mother if she could be allowed to visit me.

The second time Caroline visited me she opened up a little more and shared with me some of her concerns. What she wanted to talk to me about, and what really was her main concern, was what she felt was a structural weaknesses in her apartment that made her stay awake at nights and contributed to her worsening health. As she talked about it, she became more and more upset about the landlord who she felt knew about this but didn't do anything to fix it. So her hopes turned to me since she had the idea that I would write a letter, a medical certificate, to the landlord that would mandate him to act to improve her apartment. She told me that every night about the time when she was to go to bed, she began hearing the neighbours talking through the walls. After having complained about it for a while, she revealed to me that it was actually more the radiators than the walls that let their voices through. The voices were clearly her neighbours' voices, at least most of the time, but she could also hear other voices. She could hear the voices best when she had been lying in her bed for perhaps half an hour, relaxing, trying to sleep. Often they came very suddenly, without any warning. She was clear that it was not due to her falling asleep: she had tested this and waited for the sounds to start, and every time, they did. I asked how she could be sure about this, and I said that perhaps it still was due to her being tired. But when I said that, she abruptly interrupted me and turned her head away as if she was disappointed in me. She said, "No, no. Don't you trust me?"

I quickly tried to restore her confidence in me by stating, "Of course I do," and, "Your version is essential; it was just a routine question." She paused for a while and then (fortunately), after having gazed at the floor for a while, she continued with her story.

"The neighbours," she said, "their voices …" and then she paused again, but now having a more searching look – as if she scanned her mind for memories. "Their voices talk about me. Sometimes they are mean." The hesitation was there once more, but this time I could see her trying to fight back her angst, her fear of what she experienced.

I asked what they said, and she then looked at me with some anger in her eyes and said, "I don't want to tell you that." She then once more broke up the meeting and said she did not need any help. It all went so quickly that I had no chance of trying to convince her to stay. Suddenly, she was out of the room.

It took two days before she called me, and (as if I expected a starter phrase) she jumped immediately into her questions asking if I had written her that certificate. As we hadn't talked about the certificate at her last visit I asked about what she had in mind. She then asked me if I had forgotten. I said, "No, of course not, Caroline. It's just that you did not specify what you would like in the certificate when we last met."

"Now that's not true," she said. "How can you forget?" She was clearly upset and hung up the phone without giving me any chance to clarify or discuss the matter. I left it at that and realized that she most likely did not feel well at all and that it was clearly difficult for her to express her needs. I speculated that she was plagued by her thoughts and assumptions, and I set up a strategy to help her in the event that she called me back. In these cases, patients suffering from delusions and paranoia most commonly get very guarded and suspicious. The psychiatrist will need to work around that if he is going to help them in any way. I decided to set my ambitions and expectations low.

Interestingly, the next day I got a call from Caroline's daughter Elin who asked if she could see me. I said that she was welcome but that I needed to keep the confidentiality towards her mother, so I could not talk with her unless her mother explicitly (and preferably in writing) allowed me to share information about her. Elin accepted this and said that she was very concerned about her mother and that she only desired to speak to me and share the concern and information about her mother's health with me so that I could help Caroline in the best way. This was, of course, much appreciated, and we made an appointment for a few days later.

Elin showed up as agreed, and she looked like a spitting image of her mother – just thirty years younger –and just not tainted by thirty-five years of smoking. She had the same facial expressions and body movements as her mother. It often amazes me how much we inherit and carry forward from our forefathers/mothers in spite of our often denying it or at least trying to hide it.

Elin was a little bit hesitant at first, but she was still relaxed. It was as if she wanted me to start the conversation or perhaps that she was concerned that she would have to speak to her mother whom she knew was so paranoid. The latter turned out to be the case. We started out talking about this, and I asked how she felt about it all.

"Well," she said, "I am very concerned about my mother. On one hand she does not feel well at all and I really want to help her. On the other hand, she explicitly said to me not to speak to you about her – at least not at first. She actually yelled at me, but after a while she was more undecided. It is as if her emotions are still there – that is, the shared love we have for each other – but that the words and all other communicative signals are twisted in her brain. I had to convince her with all my love for her. It took several hours, and I am a bit exhausted by this all. Actually, I spend hours with her every time I call her or visit her. You know, she is not well at all. I am very, very concerned about her. She has lost weight, perhaps fifteen kilo, and she just can't stop smoking, either. She has ideas about the food, that it may be poisoned, and that the neighbours are trying to kill her. She thinks they try to send gas into her apartment through the radiators, so she has put tape all over all the radiators, and also on some windows, to keep gas out. This is really painful to see."

Elin stopped and looked down at the floor in front of her. I noticed how she struggled to keep the tears away. There was so much that had changed in her mother: she had struggled for years with her worsening health, both the physical and mental, and now she was close to starving herself to death – isolating herself from the threatening world outside. I gave Elin a tissue to wipe her eyes. Time passed and we sat silently for a while, allowing time to let her sadness fade a bit and let other thoughts in. Suddenly she said, "She sleeps very poorly, you know. I am not sure she sleeps at all. I have asked if she would like me to stay, but as soon as she plans to go to bed she always sends me home with an amazing and ambiguous reassurance that 'everything is all right'. It is as if she wants to (or knows that she needs to) fight her demons alone. It is heart-breaking."

She continued to talk about her mother, how she had changed, and about her concerns. We talked for an hour and then she left with a promise to herself that she would bring her mother back to me.

It took perhaps another week before Elin stood there in the doorway of the psychiatric unit holding hands with her mother. They had not made an appointment, but fortunately it was close to lunchtime so I could fit them in to my schedule. They had to wait for perhaps half an hour, and it was as if this was the final fight for Elin: she was not going to give in now that she had managed to bring her mother to the unit. Caroline looked as if she had given up; she was overly tired and worn down.

"How are you, Caroline?" I asked.

She hesitated and looked at me several times before she answered. "I am not well" she said in a weak voice.

"I can see that you are suffering, Caroline. Please tell me what I can do for you."

An even longer pause began, and I had decided to wait her out – to give her all the time she needed. Finally she responded.

"Someone is after me. I am sure of that," she said in a slow and weak voice. There are shadows everywhere I go – dark, ugly shadows. They call me. I can't stand it," she said and started to cry just a little bit, almost as if she didn't want to show it to me. She struggled with her emotions and then continued.

"The shadows are not mine, but they follow me." She looked around as if she was searching the room. "I know they are here as well."

"Caroline" I responded. "I am a physician, and there are ways that I can help to relieve you of your suffering."

She didn't react. She just looked at her daughter as if questioning why she was here and with a faint sign of a plea to her.

"They are trying to poison me", she said looking at her daughter just briefly and then turning away her gaze again towards the ground.

"Caroline," I continued. You are not well, and I will need to treat you so that you may regain your strength and health. She looked at me as if she wanted to protest, but she was too weak to ever begin. "I will prescribe you some medication that will help you," I told her. "No, no" she said. "I am not going to take any more poison. The neighbours are already after me and now you as well. Elin, what is going on? I am not ill you know. It's the neighbours."

I realized she was nowhere near any acceptance of her bad health; she did not even realize that she needed help. So, I made a decision that I knew may break our communication for a long while, but it was a medically-necessary and legally-defendable decision. I said, "Caroline, I will take you to the hospital for treatment. You are actually not well at all, and you may die if I don't take care of you".

Caroline looked at her daughter, but in vain, since her daughter looked as if she agreed with me. "Elin, what is going on? What is he trying to do? I need to go home. Elin, take me home."

After those words I started to prepare for an urgent transport to the hospital for immediate treatment. I informed Caroline and Elin what was going to happen, and Caroline complained the whole time. But by now she was so weakened by her poor sleep and starvation that she had no power to resist was what happening. A few hours later she was at the Institutional Care, a closed ward for psychoses at the local psychiatric unit. I knew the staff and the responsible physician/psychiatrist well since I had done my residency there a few years earlier. They were very good and knew exactly how they would help Caroline in the best way. This meant a combination of antipsychotic medication, daily talks and assessments, physiotherapy, good food, sleep, and high quality specialized care.

Caroline was treated for perhaps two months before she was released. I got the report that she was clearly improved and had started to accept the fact that she needed help. During her stay they had arranged for her to move to another apartment. According to Elin, some major clean-up was needed in Caroline's former apartment, but now she was to be taken care of by experienced staff that would be able to attend to her needs most of the day preventing it from going this far once more. She also got an alarm in her new apartment, and she continued her medication.

Caroline would never return to me. Although she was vastly improved, there were areas of her memory that associated me with distrust and a level of authority that she could not accept. Perhaps I was still one of those shadows that she did not want to meet ever again. That part was okay. What was important was that she did not suffer any longer, that she had regained her strength, and most importantly, that she still loved her daughter.

Caroline suffered from delusions and eventually hallucinations also. A delusion is a strong belief which is based on conviction in spite of evidence to support the contrary. It is often a symptom of a psychiatric or neurological illness. In itself, it is not a specific sign, but it can be found in several types of disorders. In Caroline's case it was due to paranoid schizophrenia, or paraphrenia. Generally, the more bizarre the delusions the more likely it is related to a psychotic disorder such as schizophrenia. In Caroline's case, it was the idea of her being poisoned and that she was followed.

Caroline was only 50 when she developed the disorder, and it may have been that the onset was triggered by a concomitant cerebrovascular disorder. The complexity of her disorder was aggravated by her lack of insight. She was completely convinced she was being poisoned and could not realize that she was ill; as such, she refused to be helped. It was the stamina, the stubbornness of her daughter and the fact that her starving depleted her of her strength that made it possible to treat her. In Caroline's case the treatment went well, but sometimes it doesn't. Fortunately there is hope. The attention to – as well as the awareness and recognition of – these disorders is increasing, and options for treatment and care are improving. My mission is to tell their stories and to spread the knowledge of psychosis and other psychiatric disorders so that more people will recognize them and learn how to help others.

THE NON-STOP LOVER

Dr. Magnus Sjögren

ABOUT THE AUTHOR

Dr Magnus Sjögren is a physician, specialist in psychiatry, a PhD and Associate Professor at the Sahlgrens University Hospital in Gothenburg, Sweden. His research is focused on clinical psychiatry, neuropsychiatry and biomarkers for disease. His inspiration for this book stems from all the fascinating patients that he has met in his work. The motivation to help, to find a cure, drove him to try to develop new medicines for difficult disorders, and he has successfully been part of research teams that made the launch of two new medicines possible. He is passionate about helping patients to find ways to improved health, and, he is enthralled about writing.

www.ingramcontent.com/pod-product-compliance
Lightning Source LLC
Chambersburg PA
CBHW051711170526
45167CB00002B/621